Health education and health promotion

Health education and health promotion

Maria A. Koelen

Anne W. van den Ban

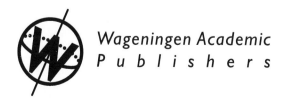

Wageningen Academic
P u b l i s h e r s

CIP-data Koninklijke Bibliotheek Den Haag

ISBN 9076998442

Subject headings:
Health related behaviour
Community action
Action and research

First published, 2004

Cover design:
Corrie Vis

Wageningen Academic Publishers

The Netherlands, 2004

Printed in The Netherlands

Acknowledgements

This book originates from the Department of Communication and Innovation Studies of Wageningen University. The Department was founded in 1964 by the second author. The first author started working at the Department in 1983 and, since then, has been dedicated to research in health promotion.

Over the years, we have observed a strongly growing interest in research into health-related issues and health promotion at our Department. Many students have dedicated their professional lives to health promotion and have found their way into interesting positions in research institutes, health promotion organisations and government bodies.

There are many books covering parts of the field, but in the course of lectures and discussions with students we felt the lack of a comprehensive book with a broad focus overseeing the field of health promotion research and practice. This brought us to the decision a couple of years ago to write a book in the tradition of another successful Wageningen textbook (65,000 copies have already been printed) that has proven to be an important source of knowledge for students and practitioners.

The book has been developed in interaction with our students at Wageningen University, students participating in the annual European courses on health promotion, and many professional friends from all over Europe. We would like to thank them all for their sincere thoughts and contributions. We have learned that health education and promotion is a field full of developments and very appealing to politicians as well as to citizens, both old and young.

Preface

Avoiding illness and promoting health has been a major concern of individuals and societies over centuries, and still is today. Achieving or improving health requires a range of actions by different agencies from social, political, economic, biomedical, behavioural, educational, environmental, and technical arenas. An increasing number of professionals, and not only health professionals, will have to play an important role in this field over the years to come.

This book provides a basic understanding of health concepts and health-related research and action programmes. It gives the reader:

- A basic understanding of the concepts of health, quality of life, disease prevention and health promotion;
- A theoretical framework for understanding, predicting and changing behavioural, social and environmental determinants of health;
- A theoretical framework for communication and communicative interventions (i.e. health education);
- A range of individual, group-oriented and population-wide strategies and actions for health education and health promotion;
- A framework for participatory action - including community participation and intersectional collaboration - and project management;
- A framework for planning, evaluation and research;
- An awareness of ethical issues relating to health promotion action and research.

It is a comprehensive resource book and a guide not only for students, scholars and practitioners, but also for policymakers, change managers, and all others who work on the promotion of health in their everyday practice. It offers a useful guide for a variety of professional and volunteer organisations and their workers, such as public health and health promotion specialists, health service managers and environmental health officers, professional and voluntary community organisations, community nurses and dieticians, midwives and paediatricians, epidemiologists and psychologists, sociologists and communication planners, dentists and dental hygienists, general practitioners and pharmacists, and social workers. The book is also suitable for all those who carry the field close to their heart and who are willing to invest in the promotion of health.

Wageningen, April 2004
Maria A. Koelen
Anne W. van den Ban

Table of contents

1. Introduction

Being healthy is a matter of importance for individuals, families, communities, and for society at large. It is generally recognised that health is essential for personal, social and economic development. The health of the population has been a matter of concern for many centuries, and it continues to be a major issue; but strategies to protect and improve health are subject to change. Until the first half of the 20th century, mortality and morbidity were strongly related to communicable diseases; for example, high mortality rates were a result of infectious diseases as well as of highly contagious (epidemic) diseases such as typhoid, tuberculosis and the plague. Medical science has provided new knowledge about diseases and their control, and it has led to advances in medicine that have been of enormous benefit to many people. Together with improvements in housing and sanitation standards, the provision of bacteriologically safe water and foods, improved living conditions, and improvements in income and education, great progress has been made in the improvement of health, especially in the last century. The demise of epidemics, declines in both maternal and infant mortality rates, and the increasing proportion of the population living into old age are just a few examples. Nevertheless, this is no time to take it easy. A large part of the world's population still suffers from ill health, and the levels of untimely mortality remain too high. New health threats emerge, due, for example, to hitherto unknown diseases and causes, but also due to environmental health threats. The disease profiles of many countries have changed remarkably in the past decades, shifting from communicable diseases to chronic, non-communicable diseases. It is estimated that non-communicable diseases account currently for approximately 60 per cent of the global disease burden.

Health is not equally distributed throughout the world. There are many differences in the health status of populations in various parts of the world, often related to economic factors. Clearly, people in industrialised nations have benefited most from economic and scientific progress. In poorer parts of the world, health risks are commonly associated with poverty, such as underweight, unsafe water, poor sanitation and hygiene, and unsafe sexual practice in relation to HIV/AIDS (WHO, 2002). Health issues are primarily related to scarcity, such as food scarcity, lack of primary health care services, lack of medicine, and lack of both human and financial resources. In industrialised parts of the world on the other hand, even though it seems contradictory, improvements in living standards have given rise to new health problems. For example, the fact that people live longer leads to an increasing number of elderly persons with their own demands on health services. More importantly however, an increasing number of health problems are related to excess and over-consumption. Morbidity and mortality rates have increased in recent decades due to health problems such as cancers, cardio-vascular diseases (including high blood pressure, high blood cholesterol), obesity, respiratory diseases (including asthma), addictions due to substance abuse (e.g. alcohol or drug abuse) and mental disorders (e.g. depression, dementia). Certainly, these health problems may be caused by biological factors, but human behaviour and the physical environment typically play a role in their development and maintenance. Moreover, economic growth, increased prosperity and increased consumption go along with increased industrial activity, placing high demands on environmental health. Hence, the improvement and sustainability of acceptable levels of health remains a major challenge. Considerable effort continues to be necessary in order to decrease mortality and morbidity and to improve both health and - in relation to this - quality of life.

However, because of such changing patterns in the causes of ill health, the actions and measures to improve and maintain reasonable levels of health are also changing. For many centuries the main burden was to cure illnesses by means of medicine, and to prevent the spread of diseases, mainly by the use of immunisation. To oversimplify: health gains were mainly achieved through the skill and dedication shown by health workers and doctors in their management of sickness, while health education was concerned with convincing people of the importance of preventive immunisation techniques and with teaching them about hygiene. In today's world, medicine alone is insufficient to combat disease and improve health. Moreover, in spite of the scientific progress in medical science, an effective cure is not yet available for several diseases. A great deal could be achieved by preventing these diseases. For example, albeit the origin of HIV/AIDS is much better understood today than 20 years ago, scientific research has not yet produced a sovereign remedy. The most effective way of controlling the spread of this communicable disease is therefore based on preventive behaviour. In addition, health is affected by a multitude of factors and by different levels in society, including individuals, families, the communities in which individuals function, organisations and health services, environmental as well as local, national and international policy levels.

Clearly, the approach to protection and improvement of health has become much wider. Treatment of established diseases remains important, but much more emphasis is needed on prevention. Besides, improving health is no longer considered to be the responsibility of the health sector alone. It involves many stakeholders from different sections in society, and includes a range of intersectoral actions by different agencies from social, political, economic and technical arenas. Advances in public health have to be achieved through a combination of structural change and actions of individuals. This is the point of departure in health promotion, the topic to be addressed in this book.

1.1 Overview of the book

Because of the above-described changes in the nature of diseases and illnesses, and also because of changes in society at large, the approach to improving the health of populations is changing. There is also change over time in the meaning of the terms health, health education, health promotion, and health policy. In order to develop a coherent and scientific view, we discuss the origins and historical development of health promotion in Chapter 2. We outline the main aims and objectives of health improvement programmes at each level, and discuss their social significance as a means to improve the quality of life.

Many health interventions are aimed at behaviour and behaviour change. A thorough knowledge of why people behave as they do is therefore an important prerequisite. In Chapter 3 we provide a theoretical background to health-related behaviour, viewed mainly from the perspective of social psychology and health psychology. We elaborate on perception and learning, and on the analysis of behaviour in terms of its determinants, such as attitudes and social influence. Behaviour change, however, does not occur overnight; rather, it is the result of processes of change. In Chapter 4 therefore, we elaborate on these processes both at the individual and the collective level, based on the adoption and diffusion of innovations theories. Most of the actions to induce individual and collective change rely on communication. In Chapter 5 we elaborate on specific features of the communication process. In Chapter 6 we present the main communication methods and discuss their strengths and weaknesses. From Chapter 7 onwards we look at the broader perspective of health promotion. The importance of the participation of target populations in health improvement programmes is increasingly acknowledged, as well as the necessity for multisectoral efforts. Hence, community participation and intersectoral collaboration are discussed in some depth in Chapter 7. In Chapter 8 we provide a framework for designing health education and health promotion programmes. Effective health education and health promotion requires sophisticated analysis of health-related problems, as well as systematic planning and evaluation. Specific attention is paid both to the analysis of health problems in terms of their behavioural and environmental causes and to the development, implementation and evaluation of comprehensive programmes. Chapter 9 deals with research into planning, implementation and evaluation.

Most professionals working in the field of health education and health promotion are associated with large or small formal organisations such as government departments, health authorities, local health services, universities or non-governmental organisations. Organisational structures and the environment in which organisations operate will have an impact on the contribution that organisations and their staff can make to health improvement. In Chapter 10 we discuss some of these issues and what they mean for individual organisations. Since health promotion often requires inter-organisational input, special attention is given to the organisation of collaborative work. Finally, influencing individual behaviour, changes in communities, and the development of policies are serious matters that may raise ethical questions. We therefore conclude the book, in Chapter 11, with ethical considerations relating to responsibilities and the nature of interventions. Finally, we discuss some of the codes of ethics that have been developed for the field.

Some of the concepts used in this book are explained in greater detail in the Glossary. We hope the readers will consult that section regularly. Health education and health promotion concerns a vast field of study encompassing many disciplines and social skills, which we cannot cover in every detail. We therefore refer readers to literature relating to these wider fields at the end of the book. Readers wishing to delve more deeply should consult the main references for further study.

2. Health, health education, health promotion and health policy

Working towards better population health is a major challenge in the 21st century. Changing patterns in health problems and in the causes of ill health urge us to consider health protection and health improvement from a broad perspective, in relation both to the issues to be addressed and to the professions and sectors involved. The importance of issues such as the reduction of stress levels, the improvement of working conditions, the availability and accessibility of health services, and the influence of environmental pollution on health is increasingly recognised. The professionals involved range from medical doctors to social workers, and from dieticians to lawyers. The sectors involved vary from health to media, industry, sports and recreation to a variety of government departments.

Together with changes in health problems and diseases, the reasoning behind *what* constitutes good health has changed, as well as the ways of considering measures to improve health. In this chapter we look at the development of the meaning of health, health education, health promotion, and health policy, by putting these concepts into an historical context. Because there are probably as many definitions of the concepts as there are workers in the field, we mostly refer to definitions provided in publications of the World Health Organisation (WHO). WHO and UNICEF are the world's largest formal agencies formulating global policy and action plans on health, which are paralleled by regional, national and local policies. Both agencies first came together in 1978 in Alma-Ata to elaborate and formulate a future global strategy for primary health care and the Health for All by the year 2000 quest. The Alma-Ata Declaration (*cf.* WHO, 1978) provided an important guide for the professional and scientific development of the field, as well as a blueprint for the development of policies in individual countries.

2.1 Health

The question 'What is health?' seems to be a simple one, but the answer is not always straightforward. In itself it is difficult to define health in terms of objective, measurable criteria. There have been many attempts to define health in meaningful ways, but opinions regarding what has to be understood by health differ across and within health care disciplines. For centuries, health was defined in terms of the absence of physical disability. From this medical-biological point of view, persons for instance suffering from chronic diseases or a physical handicap were considered to be unhealthy. It is easy to see that this definition is rather narrow, since it only incorporates physical factors, and therefore is not very useful in the field of maintaining, improving or sustaining health. An opposing position talks about personal perception and maintains that as long as individuals perceive themselves as healthy, they are healthy (e.g. Kessener, 1982). This definition is unhelpful from a theoretical point of view, as it is solely based on individual perceptions and fails to give practical cues.

Health has both objective and subjective aspects. Someone may have a disease without feeling ill, or, conversely, someone may feel ill without having a disease in the medical sense. Both of the abovementioned definitions take account of only one of these aspects. The most commonly accepted definition is that formulated in the WHO constitution of 1948: *health is a state of complete physical, social and mental wellbeing, and not merely the absence of disease or infirmity*. With this definition, health is placed in a broader context. It refers to the interaction of body and mind. Furthermore, reference is made to the importance of a positive social environment (including affectionate relationships and group membership) and to the capability of individuals to move actively within that environment. Wellbeing includes such aspects as happiness and prosperity. This view on health is in accordance with the work of Maslow (1968), a coryphaeus in humanistic psychology. Humanistic psychology emphasises the independent dignity and worth of human beings and their conscious capacity to develop personal competence and self-respect. Maslow established a hierarchy of needs, progressing from physiological needs, safety, love and esteem, to self-actualisation (see Figure 2.1). He assumed that people are motivated by unsatisfied needs and that certain lower-level needs have to be satisfied to some degree before

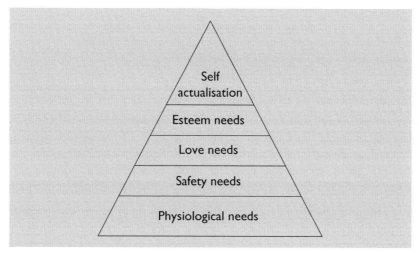

Figure 2.1 Maslow's hierarchy of needs.

higher needs can be satisfied. The basic needs relate to physiological necessities for survival (e.g. air, water, food). Safety needs have to do with establishing stability and consistency in a chaotic world (e.g. protection, security, free from threat or hazard). Love and belongingness are the next needs, and refer to feeling loved and being accepted by others. Self-esteem results from competence or mastery of a task. The need for self-actualisation refers to the desire to become everything that one is capable of, thus maximising one's potential.

It has only gradually been accepted that a person's health is influenced by many factors. These factors are generally referred to as determinants of health. We prefer to categorise them into three groups: endogenous determinants, exogenous determinants, and the prevalent system of health care (Ruwaard *et al.*, 1994).

Endogenous determinants are those that affect health 'from the inside' (see Figure 2.2). They refer to biological factors, which may be hereditary or acquired in the course of life. Gender is the first important hereditary factor. Biological differences between man and woman have different impacts on health status. For example, only women can develop cancers of the cervix, and breast cancer is almost entirely a female problem, whereas only men can develop prostate or testicular cancer. The second hereditary factor is genetic predisposition.

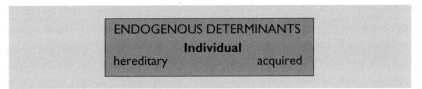

Figure 2.2 Endogenous factors influencing health.

Genetic disorders can be passed on to family members who inherit the genetic abnormality, for example some forms of cancer or colour blindness. Also, some disorders are caused by a mistake in a single gene. Acquired factors are built up in the course of life, for example, physical condition, acquired immunity, increased blood pressure, or reduced lung function as a result of an earlier infection. It should be noted that several of the endogenous determinants result from an interaction between hereditary and acquired components.

Exogenous determinants refer to external influences on health and relate to physical environment, lifestyle factors and social environment (see Figure 2.3). The physical environment includes food, hygiene and shelter, but also factors such as noise and heat, chemical factors (e.g. environmental pollution, hazardous substances in the work environment), and biotic factors (e.g. bacteria, viruses). Lifestyle factors refer to identifiable patterns of behaviour that are maintained with some consistency over time. They include conscious health-directed behaviour, but also behaviour and practices for non-health purposes that have health consequences or risks. Social environment includes socio-economic status, ethnic background, social relations and networks, working environment and housing conditions.

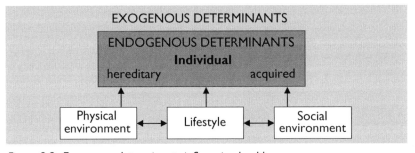

Figure 2.3 Exogenous determinants influencing health.

The third group of determinants consists of the *system of health care.* This refers to health services in relation to care, cure, and prevention. It includes diagnostic and treatment services, medical and nursing services, and health services in the arena of disease prevention and health promotion.

It is clear that the groups of determinants do not occur in isolation. They interact with each other, and together they influence the health status of individuals and populations. This is illustrated in Figure 2.4. For example, socio-economic variables such as income, education and occupation affect inactivity, diet and tobacco use, which in turn influence physical condition, increased blood pressure and cholesterol levels, to cause cardio-vascular disease or cancers.

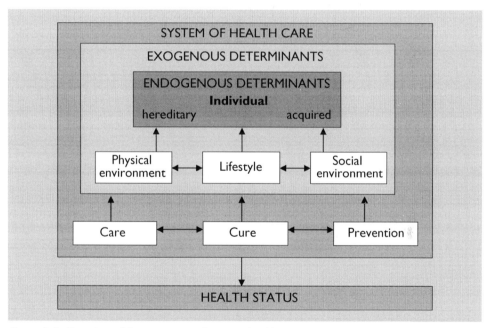

Figure 2.4 Overview of determinants influencing health.

To summarise, the conceptualisation of health has changed over the years. Whereas traditionally health was considered as an abstract state and defined in the narrow terms of absence of disease, nowadays it is looked at from a holistic point of view. It is a positive concept, expressed in functional terms. Health is not an end, but a means, a resource that enables people to lead an individually, socially and economically productive life. In this book we define health as *a state of complete physical, social and mental wellbeing, which enables people to lead an individually, socially and economically productive life.* We consider health to be interactively influenced by endogenous and exogenous determinants as well as by the system of health care.

2.2 Health education

The recognition that individual behaviour plays a pivotal role in the development and maintenance of many health problems gave momentum to the development of health education as a professional and scientific field. Amongst the major causes of mortality and morbidity are disorders such as coronary heart disease, stroke, and malignant diseases (e.g. lung-, breast-, and prostate cancer), as well as accidents in traffic and in the domestic sphere. There is ample evidence that behavioural and lifestyle factors such as diet, substance abuse (e.g. alcohol and drugs), sedentary work and leisure, and reckless behaviour contribute to the development and maintenance of these disorders. Change in such behaviours can have a major preventive and health enhancing value. In addition, individual behaviour is an essential factor in the effectiveness of medical care. For instance, a therapy (e.g. medication) will only be effective if patients comply with the therapy. A person does not keep a good set of teeth just by visiting the dentist on a regular basis; brushing teeth and low sugar consumption are also important. Traditionally, health education was based on medical practice at the time, that is, it was prescriptive and unidirectional, based on the conceptualisation of health as the absence of disease. This is also referred to as the *medical approach*. The focus was on the reduction of both morbidity and premature death. It was defined in terms of planned attempts to influence behaviour that improved the effectiveness of curative and disease-preventive interventions (see, for example, Steuart, 1965).

Health education aimed to make individuals aware of the negative consequences for health of their behaviour. The emphasis was at all times on individuals, and on single behaviours, for example 'smoking' or 'eating'. Strategies to improve health were based on helping people to form sound opinions and make good decisions. Individuals were seen as logical information processors, that is, they were expected to process that information in a logical manner and subsequently act accordingly. However, practical experiences confirmed by several studies (see Ajzen & Fishbein, 1980; Green *et al.*, 1980; Koelen, 1988) have demonstrated that, while knowledge is an important factor in inducing behaviour change, it is not in itself enough. Programmes intended to increase individuals' knowledge about health consequences of behaviour often do not lead to the expected behavioural effects, and, if an effect is found, it is usually of small magnitude. Rational cognitive appeals do not seem to possess enough power to motivate the individual to change behaviour. In general, people like doing what they do, and they do not want to change their acquired habits. Everyone knows that smoking is unhealthy and yet large numbers of people continue to puff merrily away. Motivation, skills, and perceived self-efficacy are obviously important conditions as well (e.g. Ajzen & Madden, 1986; Green & Kreuter, 1991; Bandura, 1986; see section 3.5). Moreover, much (health-related) behaviour occurs or is learnt in a social context. It is recognised that individuals cannot be isolated from their material and social context and that the function of single behaviours has to be considered in the wider context of lifestyles (Koelen, 1988).

In order to implement effective health education, the focus shifted to determinants of behaviour other than knowledge - such as social influence, skills and opportunities - and the possibility of changing such behaviour. This marked an important shift, as it considers health as the property of individuals and makes it possible to assume that people can improve their health by choosing to change their lifestyle. The approach changed to what we may call a *persuasive approach*. Individuals are encouraged to change their behaviour in a certain direction seen as conducive to health in the eyes of the expert. The aim is to provide knowledge and information, and to develop skills for individuals to make an informed choice about their health-related behaviour. Just as with the medical approach, the persuasive approach is expert-led: the expert provides the general public with education and advice to enable them to behave in a healthier manner. Likewise, it is based upon the assumption that, through an increase in knowledge, there will be changes in attitudes, which may lead to changed behaviour. Human beings, however, are not inanimate voids; they are carriers and producers of information in their own right. Information does not fall into empty minds but is integrated into what people already know and do, and into what they like and dislike. Moreover, the persuasive approach ignores the constraints that social and economic factors place on voluntary behaviour change, and also the complexities of health-related decision making. Major debates took place about the objectives of health education. Should programmes and activities aim to improve and maintain health by trying to persuade an individual to behave in a way that health professionals think is desirable, or should they try to increase an individual's capabilities of deciding for him or herself the best ways to achieve his or her goals?

Gradually, more emphasis came to be placed on gathering information from and about the intended target populations, about their opinions regarding health-related topics, about their perceived constraints towards healthy lifestyles, and also about their own notions concerning behavioural change. Hence, the approach shifted from a unidirectional one to a more interactive and participatory one. The *participatory approach* holds that health education is not a process of information transmission from the knowledgeable to the less knowledgeable, but rather a horizontal process of information exchange and interaction. In this approach, the focus is on helping people to identify their own concerns and to gain the skills and confidence to act upon those concerns. It takes into account the notion that the social and physical environment in which people live is an important factor in health. Moreover, it reflects the fact that health is no longer seen as an end in itself, but as a means to leading a productive life.

Health education today is defined as *consciously constructed opportunities for learning, involving some form of communication designed to improve health literacy, including improving knowledge, and developing life skills which are conducive to individual and community health* (WHO, 1998; Nutbeam, 1998a). This definition is interesting in that it includes the concept of health literacy. Health literacy represents the cognitive and social skills necessary to understand and use information, and to increase the confidence to take action in ways that promote and maintain good health, including changing lifestyles and living conditions. We argue that, in order to improve health literacy, organisations must take a responsible stance in their provision of information. In order to be effective, people need to have access to information and must be able to understand that information.

Furthermore we wish to emphasise the importance of participation in designing health education programmes, thus making use of the indigenous knowledge and experience of the populations involved. This is not to say that health education campaigns should never be persuasive and expert-led. Sometimes it is necessary to take such a stance, as for example when new health hazards emerge. This was the case in the early nineteen eighties with the rise of the HIV/AIDS epidemic. For many other issues however, active involvement of the target groups themselves is the most desirable approach. We therefore slightly rephrase the definition of health education as: consciously constructed opportunities for learning, *together with (representatives of) the target population*, involving some form of communication designed to improve health literacy, including improving knowledge, and developing life skills which are conducive to individual and community health.

2.3 Health promotion

Health education focuses on influencing and changing individual behaviour. However, health is affected by endogenous factors, exogenous factors, and the health care system. Recognition of the interaction of these elements had consequences for what are considered appropriate actions to promote positive health. It became evident that the achievement of health could not be the responsibility of the health care sector alone. In order to tackle health problems, a broader approach is necessary, addressing both the endogenous and exogenous determinants of health as well as the system of health care. A new concept emerged, the concept of health promotion. At the first International Conference of Health Promotion in Ottawa, 1986, a Charter was presented (WHO, 1986), which describes health promotion as *the process of enabling individuals and communities to increase control over, and to improve their health*. Health education is still considered to be an important device for the improvement of health, but, as Kickbush (1986) states, it can only develop its full potential if it is supported by structural measures such as legal, environmental, and regulatory ones. For example, in health education, much attention has been paid to the health consequences of smoking. One can observe a general decrease in the number of smokers in industrialised countries since the 1960s. In The Netherlands, for instance, the number of smokers decreased from about 80 per cent of the male population and 30 per cent of the female population in the sixties to 35 per cent for both males and females today. It is quite apparent that factors other than health education have brought this about, such as legislative measures that obliged the industry to warn smokers about the health consequences. Furthermore, measures such as the prohibition of smoking in public places, trains and planes have contributed, as have increased taxes on tobacco.

Health promotion thus involves a broader area of action than health education alone. Whereas health education focuses on individual behaviour, health promotion takes into account the broader context. This becomes very clear if we consider the five principles on which health promotion is based (Ashton & Seymour, 1988). These are: (1) health promotion actively involves the population in everyday-life settings; (2) it is directed towards action on the causes of ill health; (3) it uses many different approaches; (4) it depends particularly on public participation; and (5) health professionals have an important part to play in nurturing health promotion. We will elaborate further on each principle.

Involving populations
Health promotion actively involves the population in everyday-life settings. This principle contains two important elements. Firstly, it shows that the focus is on *populations* instead of on individual behaviour. Many health problems nowadays are seen as being social rather than solely individual problems. Secondly, it considers the notion of *settings*. 'Settings' refers to the place or social context in which people engage in daily activities, and in which environmental, organisational and personal factors interactively affect health and wellbeing (*cf.* Nutbeam, 1998a). This can be the neighbourhood in which people live, schools, workplaces and places to spend leisure time, hospitals, or cities. They are those places in which people live, act and interact with the social and physical environment, and which can have a positive or negative impact on people's health.

Action on causes of ill health
The second principle states that health promotion is directed towards action on the *causes* of ill health. This means that the focus is on prevention rather than on cure, but it also recognises the necessity of

a broad approach, that is, that action should be directed at the social and physical environment. In this sense it resembles one of the action points of the Ottawa Charter (WHO, 1986), i.e. create a supportive environment. People live their lives in the larger environment. Several conditions in the environment can be a cause of ill health. A supportive environment includes living and working conditions that are safe, stimulating, satisfying and enjoyable. Furthermore, it aims at the protection of the natural and built environments and the conservation of natural resources. Thus, health promotion aims to create environments that support people to lead an individually, socially and economically healthy and productive life.

Different approaches

Thirdly, health promotion uses many different approaches, including education and information, community development and organisation, health advocacy and legislation. Two action points in the Ottawa Charter (WHO, 1986) refer to this. (1) Develop *personal skills*. Health promotion should support personal and social development through providing information and education. By doing so, it increases the options available to people in making informed choices conducive to health. Furthermore, enhancing life skills facilitates the opportunities for people to exercise more control over their own health and over their environment. Enabling people to learn throughout life, to prepare themselves for all of its stages, and to cope with chronic illness and injuries is essential. This can be facilitated in school, home, work and community settings. (2) Build *public policies* that support health. This includes, amongst other things, the notion that health has to be on the agenda of policy makers in all sectors and at all levels, directing them to be aware of the health consequences of their decisions and to accept their responsibilities for health. The aim must be to make the healthier choice the easier choice.

Public participation

Fourthly, health promotion depends particularly on public participation. This point refers to the notion of community participation. We use the term 'community' to refer to specific groups with shared living needs, shared values, interests, cultural patterns and social problems. This can apply to groups living in a certain geographical area, but also to groups such as those found in schools or workplaces (see settings). Community participation means that health promotion is carried out by people and with people, and must not be confused with a regime imposed from above. People actively participate in the identification of their needs, setting priorities, taking decisions, and planning strategies and implementing them in order to meet these needs. Such participation improves the capacity of groups, organisations, or communities to influence the determinants of health. It facilitates mobilisation for action and generates a sense of ownership. This relates to the action point in the Ottawa Charter (WHO, 1986) exhorting the strengthening of community action. At the heart of this process is the empowerment of communities, their ownership and control of their own endeavours and destinies. Community development draws on existing human and material resources in the community to enhance self-help and social support. A prerequisite for community action is that its members have full and continuous access to information, learning opportunities, and funding support. If these community development initiatives are starved of funds they will be like flowers starved of water - they will not bloom.

The role of health professionals
Fifthly, health professionals have an important part to play in nurturing health promotion and enabling it to take place. The Ottawa Charter (WHO, 1986) refers to this point as re-orienting health services. The role of the health sector needs to move increasingly in the health promotion direction, beyond its responsibility for providing clinical and curative services. The consequence of this is two-fold. It requires not only a change of attitude on the part of professionals, but also a change in the organisation of health services. Even though the importance of participatory approaches is recognised, the downstream transfer of information (from the professionals to the public) is dominant over the upstream transfer of information (from the public to the professionals). This may seem contradictory to what we said earlier about the shift from a unidirectional approach to a more participatory approach, but it is not. The shift mainly reflects the intention to take the characteristics of the target population into account. In fact it is not surprising, since professionals are educated to be experts and trained in top-down approaches. In the provision of their - often specialised - service, organisations have the tendency to look at individuals from that specialist point of view. This is not to say that all organisations providing health services should offer wide-ranging services, but that they should refocus on the needs of the individual as a whole person.

They have a shared responsibility. Health service institutions and governments must work together towards a health care system that contributes to the pursuit of health.

In the description of the five principles, the concept of intersectoral collaboration is interwoven. Intersectoral collaboration, also referred to as intersectoral action or intersectoral work, refers to a means of working together (collaboration) between sectors at all levels of governance and society. These sectors could be, for example, environment, transport, agriculture, food industry, housing, church, community groups and media professionals, and they may involve both professionals and non-professionals. Intersectoral collaboration has the potential for synergy. It means that many people, representing different institutions, with different backgrounds, different expertise and qualities, co-operate to achieve goals that they are unable to reach independently.

To summarise, health promotion brings together actions directed at strengthening the skills and capabilities of individuals, and actions directed towards changing social, environmental and economic conditions that may have an impact on public and individual health. Health education still has a central place but it is realised that, in order to be successful, it has to be supported by organisational, policy, and regulatory measures. Moreover, the population itself should be actively involved. What is needed is an interactional approach, with active sharing of information, dialogue with the target population, and participation in decision making. Therefore, individual and community participation and intersectoral collaboration are key principles. Health promotion is the responsibility of governments, of organisations working in the health sector, and of other sectors that affect health.

2.4 Health policies

Health promotion is based on health policy. *Policy* refers to the set of objectives and rules guiding the activities of an organisation or an administration. *Healthy public policies* means policies in the many and diverse fields which support the promotion of health. Health policy thus defines priorities and parameters for action in response to health needs, available resources, and other political pressures. It also covers the actions of governments and other institutions that are aimed at maintaining and improving the health of the population. A distinction can be made between prevention policy, health care policy, and intersectoral policy (*cf.* Ruwaard *et al*, 1994). *Prevention policy* is concerned with measures and activities aiming to prevent health problems. Prevention is generally divided into three types: primary, secondary, and tertiary. *Primary prevention* aims to prevent health problems, diseases and accidents before they occur. It refers to actions undertaken to affect or remove the risk factors conducive to disease and disorders in an entire population or specific groups at risk. Examples are vaccination for infectious diseases, and interventions aiming to influence behaviour and lifestyles conducive to health. It should be noted that primary prevention is only possible when causes are known and preventive strategies are available and feasible. When causes are unknown, or when preventive strategies are not feasible, early diagnosis and treatment of disease and disorders are important. This is the focus of *secondary prevention,* which aims to limit the course of a disease or to reduce the risk of recurrence. Screening of at-risk groups for hypertension, screening of women between 30 and 60 for breast or cervical cancer, and six-monthly dental check-ups are examples. *Tertiary prevention* aims to prevent existing health problems becoming worse, and to reduce disability due to health problems. It includes treatment and therapy, but also counselling to help patients to cope with the new - disabled - situation.

Regardless of the type, preventive action includes the promotion of lifestyles conducive to health, prevention of preventable conditions, rehabilitation, and accessible and affordable health services. Strategies may include giving information, education and training, treatment and therapy; improving conditions that otherwise give rise to disease, such as environmental pollution, traffic hazards and poor working conditions; and legislation and public policies. It may involve collective measures to prevent specific diseases, that is, *disease prevention* (e.g. vaccination or screening programmes); measures to reduce the influence of harmful factors at home and at work, that is, *health protection*; and measures to promote health, thus, *health promotion* (e.g. information and education) and measures to protect health (e.g. regulations on safety).

As mentioned above, as well as prevention policy, two additional policy areas are distinguished. *Health care policy* is concerned with (the organisation of) diagnostics, treatment, nursing and care. *Intersectoral policy* refers to policy that lies outside the strict public health sphere but still involves the prevention of damage to health, such as agricultural policy, and policy on road safety. Those policies exist either at local or national level, and most often are based on WHO policy. We will, therefore, in the next section spell out this WHO policy.

2.4.1 WHO policy

In 1977, the World Health Assembly decided that the major social goal of governments and WHO should be the attainment by all people of the world by the year 2000 of a level of health that would permit them to lead a socially and economically productive life. In 1981, the Assembly unanimously adopted a Global Strategy for Health for All by the Year 2000. According to this strategy, the task was to ensure that by the year 2000 'all people in all countries should have at least such a level of health that they are capable of working productively and of participating actively in the social life of the community in which they live' (WHO, 1981). According to the WHO, 'Health for All' does not mean an end to disease and disability, or that doctors and nurses will care for everyone. It means that resources for health are evenly distributed and that essential health care is accessible to everyone. It means that health begins at home, in schools, and in the workplace, and that people use better approaches for preventing illness and alleviating unavoidable disease and disability. It means that people recognise that ill health is not inevitable and that they can shape their own lives and the lives of their families free from the avoidable burden of disease. Three main objectives were identified:

- *The promotion of lifestyles conducive to health*, including the development of individual awareness of health risks, improvement of social and economic conditions that influence the choice of lifestyle, reduction of self-imposed health risks (e.g. alcohol and other drug dependencies, sexually transmitted diseases) by information and education but also legislative and regulatory controls.
- *Prevention of preventable conditions*, amongst which are provision of adequate primary care, reduction of communicable diseases, reduction of accidents, encouragement of balanced nutrition, and the provision of safe water and sanitation.

- *Rehabilitation and health services,* including access to community-based primary health care, special services for underserved and high-risk groups (e.g. elderly, handicapped), earlier diagnosis and intervention to prevent chronic and degenerative disease, improvements in the quality and cost effectiveness of services as well as in the equity of provision.

The underlying intention of the strategy was that each country and region within countries should develop their own Health for All strategy. Within Europe, the WHO Regional Office has further developed this objective in its own strategy, and all member states have agreed on 38 regional Health for All targets (WHO Europe, 1981). Clearly, the objective that 'by the year 2000 all people in all countries should have at least such a level of health that they are capable of working productively and of participating actively in the social life of the community in which they live' was an over-ambitious one. A great deal still needs to be done to achieve this goal, if it is possible at all. Despite this, Health for All provides a comprehensive framework for health improvement and has had a major impact on health development both globally and in Europe. In 1994, WHO's member states acknowledged that significant global changes had occurred since the introduction of Health for All, and they called for a renewal of the strategy at the dawn of the 21st century. In May 1998 all WHO member states adopted the policy of 'Health for All in the 21st century' (WHO, 1998). It sets out global priorities for the first two decades of the 21st century and aims to create the necessary conditions for people throughout the world to reach and maintain the highest attainable level of health.

The European Region of WHO refined the previous 38 targets 'in the light of past achievements and new challenges' and defined 21 targets for the 21st century, which together make up the essence of regional policy. Table 2.1 gives an overview.

These targets are clustered into five groups, and together provide a framework for the construction of targets at national and local levels. The first group, *solidarity and equity in health* (1 - 2), attempts to foster stronger equity and solidarity in health development between member states of the region and better equity and solidarity in health among groups within each country. It is based on the notion that poverty is a major cause of ill health. The better off live several years longer and

Table 2.1 Focus of the 21 targets for the 21sth century of WHO European Region.

Targets 1-2: Solidarity and equity in health

1. Solidarity for health in the European region
2. Equity in health

Targets 3-9: Better health for the people of the European Region   ‾

3. Healthy start in life
4. Health of young people
5. Healthy aging
6. Improving mental health
7. Reducing communicable diseases
8. Reducing noncummunicable diseases
9. Reducing injury from violence and accidents

Targets 10-14: Multi sectoral strategy for sustainable health

10. A healthy and safe physical environment
11. Healthier living
12. Reducing harm from alcohol, drugs and tobacco
13. Settings for health
14. Multisectoral responsibility for health

Targets 15-18: Changing the focus: an outcome oriented health sector

15. An integrated health sector
16. Managing for quality of care
17. Funding health services and allocating resources
18. Developing human resources for health

Targets 19-21: Managing change for health

19. Research and knowledge for health
20. Mobilising partners for health
21. Policies and strategies for health for all.

have fewer illnesses and disabilities than the poor. The second group, *better health for the people of WHO's European Region* (3-9), addresses the strengthening of health throughout life, and the reduction of the incidence and prevalence of diseases and other causes of ill health or death to the lowest feasible levels. The third group, a *multisectoral strategy for sustainable health* (10-14), is based on the notion that health improvement is not up to the health sector alone. It aims to create sustainable health through more health-promoting physical, economic, social and cultural environments for people. The fourth group, *changing the focus: an outcome oriented health sector* (15 - 18), is meant to orient the health sector towards ensuring better health gain, equity and cost-effectiveness. Finally, the fifth group, *managing change for health* (19-21), aims to create a broad societal movement for health through innovative partnerships, unifying policies, and management practices tailored to the new realities of Europe.

WHO health policy covers each of the policy areas we described in the previous section, that is prevention policy, health care policy, and intersectoral policy. The member states are expected to translate the targets into their own national health policies. The focus of the national policies will be slightly different, due to the differences in the health status of their populations.

2.5 Chapter summary

In this chapter we defined the concepts of health, health education, health promotion, and health policy. We described how the conceptualisation of health has changed over time and, as a consequence, the conceptualisation of how to maintain or enhance the health of individuals and populations. This also becomes obvious in the different approaches used to promote health. There is a shift away from an individual focus to a more social one, as well as from a prescriptive top-down way of working to a more participatory approach. Due to the complexity of health and the variety of factors influencing it, health education programmes and health promotion activities have to be based on a broad perspective, taking into account each of the abovementioned determinants.

3. Theoretical background to health behaviour

Many diseases are related to the way in which people behave and take care of their own health. The promotion of behaviours conducive to health therefore is one of the central arenas for action with regard to health improvement. However, it is one thing to know that a particular behaviour negatively affects health, but quite another to know how to change such behaviour. In this chapter we address theories that are important for understanding why people behave as they do. We follow the route of the individual as a learner to the individual as a social being. First we describe some general characteristics of perception. Since many of the things people do or think are the result of learning processes, we elaborate on learning, and on the ways people try to *explain* and *understand* the things they perceive. We then continue with theories that describe behaviour in terms of its underlying determinants, and we elaborate on theories that deal with the function of attitudes, subjective norms, self-efficacy and fear. In addition, since health-related behaviour quite often has social functions, we also discuss social influence and group processes.

3.1 Perception

Perception is the process by which individuals receive information or stimuli from their environment and transform it into psychological awareness. Although people live in the same world and receive similar impressions of it through their eyes and ears, and to a lesser extent through the senses of touch, taste and smell, they interpret their experiences differently. These differences in interpretation can be understood if we consider some general principles of perception.

Firstly, *perceptions are relative* rather than absolute. Although we may not be able to judge the exact weight or surface area of an object, we may be able to tell whether it is heavier or lighter, or larger or smaller than another similar object. When we first enter a darkened room during the screening of a film, we will see only the image on the screen and the bright light from the projector. After a minute or so, we will be able to see other people in the room. In other words, initial perception of darkness in the room is relative to the amount of light outside. Perception is also influenced by the surroundings of the perceived stimuli. A circle surrounded by larger circles will look smaller than a circle of the same size surrounded by smaller circles.

Secondly, *perceptions are selective*. Our senses continuously receive a veritable flood of stimuli from the environment around us. We see objects, hear noises, smell odours and so on. Despite its capacity to process vast amounts of information, the nervous system cannot make sense of all the stimuli available. Hence, an individual pays attention only to a selection of these stimuli. Selectivity is influenced by several physical and psychological factors, including attitudes. We discuss selective processes in greater detail in section 5.4.

Thirdly, *perceptions are organised*. People tend to structure their sensory experiences in ways that make sense to them. We try to convert the 'booming, buzzing confusion' into some meaningful order. One form of organisation is into *figure and ground*. In a fraction of a second, our senses sort out visual and oral stimuli in figures that stand out from a background. The interpretation of the 'figure' will often be determined by the 'ground'. One might interpret a picture of a man with a dirty face and hands and wearing old clothes as a lazy or very poor person. On the other hand, one might interpret the picture as one of a hard-working farmer, if it included a farmyard in the background. The figure and ground effect is shown in Figure 3.1.

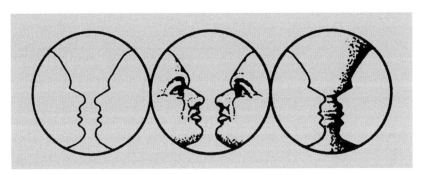

Figure 3.1 Figure and ground

Interpretations of what we perceive are often based on experiences. People have a natural tendency to form generalisations - concepts and categories that represent an oversimplification of the stimuli around us. They are stored in memory, in the form of 'mental sets'. Based on these categorisations we recognise some sorts of object as belonging to a certain category (for example, a long thing can be identified as a pencil) and next to it add certain characteristics (e.g. I can write with this pencil, without first having tried it). Categorisation helps us to find a way through the overwhelming number of stimuli from the environment. It enables us to 'type' a single event, place it in a familiar rubric, and act accordingly. For example, if we see that the sky is getting dark during the day, we assume that it is going to rain, and adjust to this situation by taking an umbrella with us if we go out. Perceptual set may also be a major deterrent, especially in situations in which it is important to interpret the situation in a new way. People tend to respond to stimuli through habit, and these habitual responses must be broken if we are to perceive a situation in a new way. This is a common problem, for example, if we work with people from different cultural backgrounds. Experience in India has shown that rural people often have difficulty understanding Western style paintings, because they use a quite different visual code from the religious paintings they are used to in their temples. Equally, Westerners often find these religious paintings difficult to interpret.

3.2 Learning

Learning is basic to human behaviour and it is a continuing part of life. Learning begins as soon as one is born (some argue that it begins before birth) and continues throughout life. The acquisition of knowledge and the development of understanding are essential parts of the learning process. Much research has been conducted into learning, but there is as yet no integrated or generally accepted theory. We restrict our discussion to some of the general principles about how people learn. As there are many sources and methods for learning, it is not easy to give a general definition of learning. Here we define learning as *acquiring or improving the ability to perform a behaviour pattern through experience and practice.* This definition is stated in terms of behaviour, and it implies a norm for the behavioural pattern at which we are aiming. If one is learning to swim, the aim may be to swim further, to swim faster or to improve swimming style. Learning can also be defined in terms of 'acquiring or improving a cognitive pattern'. However, it is difficult to know whether the cognitive pattern has changed unless the learner has shown it in some form of behaviour, for example in a verbal expression. 'The ability to perform' is included in the definition, because much learning is aimed at changing cognitions that can be used to change behaviour some time in the future. In our opinion, learning has already taken place at the moment these cognitions change. 'Through experience and practice' has been added to distinguish the process from changes caused by biological growth.

3.2.1 The Law of Effect

A basic law of learning is the Law of Effect, that is: 'an action which leads to a desirable outcome is likely to be repeated in similar circumstances'. We purposely use the phrase 'leads to' and not 'is followed by', because we consider the process of thinking about relations between cause and effect as essential in learning (see also section 3.3). If a group of people pray for rain and a rain shower follows this action, some might think that the prayers have led to the rain, whereas others may think that the rainfall was accidental. Only the first group is convinced that they should pray for rain again during the next drought. In the Law of Effect approach, it is assumed that learning is an associative process that can take place without active thinking. This is also called 'the stimulus-response model'. Famous researchers in this area are Pavlov (classical conditioning; Pavlov's dog) and Skinner (operant conditioning; the Skinner box).

A central concept in the Law of Effect is reinforcement. Reinforcement can be defined as *any event whose occurrence increases the probability that a stimulus will on subsequent occasions evoke a response* (Hilgard *et al.*, 1975). Two types of reinforcers can be distinguished: *positive reinforcers* (such as food), which increase the probability of a response, and *negative reinforcers* (such as spanking), which decrease the probability of a response. Generally, acts that lead to rewards are likely to be repeated, whereas acts leading to punishments are less likely to recur. What constitutes a reward or a punishment depends on a person's social environment, on experience in the past, and probably also on personality. Food is usually a reward, but perhaps not if politeness has already compelled you to eat more than you intended. It can be particularly rewarding if we have been able to solve a problem that we could not solve in the past. Success, therefore, is also a reward. It should be noted that rewards are more effective than punishments. For example, for a person trying to lose weight it is rewarding to see the pointer on the scale slowly going down. This reward encourages the person to continue the diet. On the other hand, a person who receives a fine because of ignoring the speed limit while driving will probably drive carefully the next day, but speed up again the following day. Rewards and punishments are not just physical or financial. They are often social in nature as well, that is, when a person's action is rewarded by another person's response. Recognition by others, being accepted, and gaining support are examples of social rewards. Rejection by others or disapproval are examples of social punishments.

3.2.2 Vicarious learning

Learning does not result only from direct - personal - experience and one's own actions. Behaviour is often learned from *observing* the actions of others and the consequences of those actions. In his social learning theory, Bandura (1977; 1986) refers to this as vicarious learning or modelling. In contrast to the stimulus-response approach, Bandura takes a cognitive viewpoint into account for learning and behaviour. He argues that people only can learn when they are aware of *what* is being reinforced, and subsequently think about and interpret these experiences. Vicarious learning thus is a cognitive process. Vicarious learning is affected by several variables, but most important are the observed consequences of the model's behaviour and the characteristics of the model. If the *consequences* of the observed behaviour are positive, the observer is likely to imitate and repeat the behaviour of the model; if the consequences are negative, the observer is likely not to imitate the behaviour. It is important to note, however, that vicarious learning occurs without reinforcement. Rewards are gained indirectly. Observers see that the modelled behaviour is rewarded and imagine themselves in the exact situation with the same outcome. This is called vicarious reinforcement. With regard to the *characteristics of the model*, it is generally agreed that people learn more from models that are competent, attractive, likable, admired and loved. The model can be a peer, a teacher, a parent, a sports celebrity, a movie star, or even a cartoon character. However, the similarity of the model plays a role. If an observer sees two models doing two different things, the observer usually learns more from the model who is similar to the observer. Modelling is applied in such diverse behaviours as fear response, aggression, skills, assertiveness, and ways to overcome phobias. Modelling is often used in the advertising field, for example, to show consumers how to use products (from washing powder to perfumes and cars) and at the same time show the product in an ideal setting for the observer; but modelling can also be used to influence health-related behaviour, both to strengthen desired, and to inhibit undesired, responses.

3.2.3 Cognitive map

Learning is not a process wherein responses are regulated solely by their immediate consequences, without requiring conscious involvement of the individual. As Bandura (1977) argues, cognitive processes play a prominent role in the acquisition and retention of new behaviour patterns. Transitory experiences leave lasting effects by being coded and retained in symbols for memory representation. Bruner (1966) refers to this representation as the *cognitive map*. This map is constructed by observing objects and events (including one's own and other people's behaviour), analysing the observations, and then making generalisations from this analysis. The process of constructing a cognitive map is basically the same as a scientific research process. Bruner assumes that it is not that important to teach children a lot of facts in schools. It is more useful for them to learn to discover relationships between facts and phenomena. Therefore, teachers try to structure what is already known, as well as new information, in such a way that children gain new insights after having spent some time trying to solve a problem. This breakthrough often does not take place at the moment of problem solving, but some time afterwards when one is not working on any particular problem. It happens after one thinks about relevant information when trying to solve the problem in question. Thus it is a way of changing a person's cognitive map of reality.

To summarise, influencing or changing the pattern of rewards and punishments can stimulate learning. Learning also occurs through observation of others. On the other hand, these cognitions can be changed through an active process of thinking. This process is stimulated by the learner's motivation to solve a certain problem, by a clear structure of the information needed to solve it, and by several attempts to apply this information to finding a solution for a problem.

3.3 Attribution

The process of thinking about relations between cause and effect is essential in learning. This is also the issue in attribution theory. Attribution theory is concerned with the way in which people try to *explain* and *understand* events. The basic assumption is that individuals are motivated to live in a meaningful and structured world. Given this motive, they are seldom - or seldom content to be - passive observers of events, but are actively involved in understanding the events they observe. Suppose you are in your room, reading a book, when suddenly the door opens (event). You will immediately stop reading and look up from the book, wondering what is happening. Why is the door opening? What is the cause of the event? You will try to understand what has happened, try to find an explanation. Did the door open because of a sudden storm, or is someone coming in? Or is there another reason (cause)? Practically, you make a cause-effect analysis. Thus, individuals interpret events and experiences in terms of their causes. These interpretations play an important role in determining reactions to such events and experiences. Ascribing an effect to a cause is called *causal attribution*. Causal attributions are important determinants of a person's interaction with the world (Kelley & Michela, 1980). The process of attribution is important to explain observed events, to predict future events, and to be able to anticipate them. The aim is to arrive at veridical causal judgements, and to encourage and maintain effective exercise of control (Kelley, 1967; 1973; Försterling, 1986; Van Knippenberg & Koelen, 1985). A proper understanding of the causes of events fosters adequate action, or, in Kelley's (1973) words, the person undoubtedly fares better in his or her decisions and actions than he or she would in the absence of the causal analysis.

Attribution theorists are guided by the belief that individuals use cognitive schemata by which they rationally process the available information, and that they use 'naive' scientific methods. Kelley (1967; 1973) describes the rules that an observer uses to make attributions of causality, either for his or her own or for another person's responses to events. Central in this is the principle of co-variation. This principle states that 'An effect is attributed to one of its possible causes with which, over time, it co-varies' (Kelley, 1973:108). In other words, the cause will be attributed to the stimulus, which is present if the event occurs and which is absent if the event does not occur. For example, you are walking along the street and suddenly you begin to get wet. You look up and see that it has started to rain. You will attribute the cause of getting wet (event) to the stimulus - rain. Causes of events can be attributed either to the observed person (to recall, this can be oneself, or another observed person) or to aspects external to the person. The latter category includes other persons or other environmental circumstances. Attribution to the person is called *internal attribution*; attribution to environmental causes is called *external attribution*.

3.3.1 Dimensions of information

According to the theory, individuals may use three dimensions of information in trying to explain and understand cause-effect relations: the entity dimension, the consensus dimension, and the time/modality dimension (Kelley, 1967; 1973). The *entity* dimension contains the stimuli that elicit the response. This dimension gives information about the *distinctiveness* of a response. A response is distinctive if the individual does not respond to all entities in the way he or she responds to the current one. For example, a girl laughs if she sees one clown (entity), but not if she sees other clowns. If the response is distinctive, the cause of the girl's laughter is attributed to the entity, in this case the clown, and thus it is an external attribution. The *consensus* dimension includes the observed actor together with other persons. A response is consensual if others react to the entity in the same way as the individual. Hence, if others also laugh when they see the specific clown, the response is consensual. In this situation, the cause is attributed to the clown. However, if the girl is the only one laughing, there is no consensus; the cause is attributed to the girl we observe, and thus the attribution is internal. The *time/modality* dimension includes the time and context in which the response occurred. This dimension gives information about the *consistency* of the response. A response is consistent if the individual responds to the entity in the same way at different times and in different modalities. So, if the girl always laughs when she sees the specific clown, regardless of whether she sees the clown on television or in the circus, her response is consistent. Consistent responses are typically ascribed to the person, that is, internally attributed.

Several studies have shown that individuals indeed make use of the three information dimensions in inferring causes of events. However, in general, consistency information has the strongest effect on causal attributions, especially in relation to the attribution of performances (e.g. Orvis *et al.*, 1975; Hewstone & Jaspers, 1983). It is specifically for this reason that attribution theory is interesting for health-related behaviour. The process of making causal attributions aims to encourage and maintain feelings of control. Causes that are attributed internally are under the control of an individual, whereas causes attributed to external factors are outside the control of the individual. For example, someone who was involved in a car accident will try to explain how this accident was caused. If he attributes the cause internally (e.g. I was driving too fast; I was not paying attention to the other traffic), the person can think about actions to prevent similar accidents in the future. Thus, he will regain control. If attribution of the cause is to factors outside, thus an external attribution (e.g. the other person was not paying attention to the traffic; the road was slippery), this will leave the person with serious doubts as to how to prevent similar accidents. Other people and slippery roads are typically outside the individual's control. There is a fair chance that the person will participate in traffic again more comfortably after internal rather than external attributions.

3.3.2 Dimensions of causality

The value of attribution theory becomes more apparent if we consider the model as developed by Weiner *et al.* (1971), who elaborate further on internal and external attributions of causality. An event or outcome is not necessarily perceived to be caused by one factor; rather, several causes may be responsible. Consider a person failing to lose weight. This person may attribute his or her failure, for example, to a lack of ability to stick to a diet, to not having tried hard enough, to metabolism, or to special circumstances such as holidays. Attributing the cause of failure to lose weight to the inability to stick to a diet or to not putting in enough effort are examples of internal attribution: both are under the control of the individual. Attributing the cause to metabolism or holidays are examples of external attributions, but there are important differences in these causes as to the extent to which they are changeable. Weiner *et al* (1971) recognised the importance of this, and added a second dimension of causality, the so-called *stability* dimension. This dimension indicates the extent to which a cause is changeable over time. For internal attribution, ability for instance may be considered relatively stable over time, whereas effort can be seen as fluctuating and thus unstable. With regard to external attributions, metabolism is rather stable. Weiner refers to this as task difficulty. Holidays on the other hand are incidental, and therefore this is an unstable cause, referred to as luck. The stability of the attribution influences the expectation of success. A person who attributes failure to stable causes is likely to expect failure again next time, because it is likely that these causes will not have changed when he or she attempts to perform the same task again. A person who attributes failure to an unstable cause might expect success next time, because the cause has perhaps changed. Consistency of information plays an important role in these attributions. Consistency in performance, thus consistency over time and modality of both success and failure, most often evoke stable internal attributions, more specifically attributions to ability or lack of ability. Inconsistency in performance may lead to unstable internal attribution (effort), but most often it leads to external attributions such as task difficulty or luck. The dimensions are illustrated in Figure 3.2.

According to Weiner (1986), people react differently to an event if they attribute the event to different causes. Perceived causes of an outcome determine a person's reactions when the same task has to be repeated. We have already mentioned that internal attributions enhance a person's feeling of control. A person will feel more confident about success if success is internally attributed than if it is attributed to external causes. This effect is intensified when the cause is stable. Confidence will be stronger if the internal cause is stable (i.e. ability)

	Stable	Unstable
Internal	ability	effort
External	task difficulty	luck

Figure 3.2 Dimensions of causality and resulting attributions.

than if the cause is unstable (effort). Consistent failure in a task, for example losing weight, leads to stable internal attribution (lack of ability) and therefore reduces confidence. Lowered success expectancies will lead individuals to think it is inefficient to invest a lot of energy in the task, because they think they may not succeed.

It should be noted that the theory deals with the way individuals actually derive causes from consequences and not how they *ought* to make such derivations. This means that attributions are subjective, but also that they can be changed. This is especially important in the case of failure. Attributions most vulnerable to change are the internal unstable attributions: they are relatively easily changeable and under personal control. Attributions less vulnerable to change are the external stable attributions. For example, attributing failure to lose weight to a lack of effort can induce a person to put in some extra effort next time. Attributing the same failure to metabolism will discourage the person from taking any action because it is a stable cause, out of his or her own control. During the past 30 years, considerable attention has been devoted to so-called reattribution programmes. Reattribution programmes try to help people to explain their performance in such a way that an attribution is made which ensures confidence and feelings of control. This includes helping people to see their own influence on a performance, and to increase feelings of confidence. A step-by-step approach is common in reattribution programmes, initially setting targets that are easy to reach. For example, an obese person may have to lose up to 30 kg of weight. This is a high target, and usually the person will not succeed. This will increase the feeling of loss of control. Therefore, it would be more helpful for the person to have targets set that are easier to reach, e.g. an initial weight loss of five kg. This increases the chance of success, which increases the motivation to continue, especially if successes are followed up by additional successes. The most important thing is that individuals feel that certain outcomes are under their personal control. Feelings of control increase self-confidence, and therefore they increase the chance that an individual will persist in that behaviour. Reattribution programmes have successfully been applied in a variety of settings: for example in the field of clinical psychology (e.g. Försterling, 1986; 1988), psychiatry (e.g. Brewin, 1985), recovery processes after accidents and coping with handicaps (e.g. Brewin, 1982; Rogner & Frey, 1985) and school performances (Siero, 1987); but also in relation to specific health risk behaviours, such as smoking (*cf.* Eiser & Van Der Pligt, 1986) and weight management (*cf.* Haish *et al.*, 1985). These studies show that reattribution can help people to increase their confidence, and consequently their performance.

3.4 Attitudes

The concept of attitude has played a major role in psychology for many decades. For a long time it has been assumed that attitude was the best predictor of behaviour. Krech, Crutchfield and Ballachey (1962:139) argue, 'Man's social actions - whether these actions involve religious behaviour, ways of earning a living, political activity, or buying and selling goods - are directed by his attitude'. But what is an attitude?

An attitude can be defined as a relatively enduring tendency to respond to an object in a way that reflects a positive or negative evaluation of that object. An attitude object can be another person, a thing (e.g. a car, a specific brand of coffee), or a specific behaviour (e.g. reduction of fat intake, condom use). A person's attitude towards a specific object has consequences for how he or she will act vis-à-vis that object. Eagly and Chaiken (1993) distinguish three types of responses: cognitive, affective and behavioural. To explain these responses, consider the example of condom use. Cognitive responses are expressions of *beliefs* about the attitude object, for example the belief that using a condom will prevent infection with HIV. Affective responses are expressions of *feelings* towards the attitude object, for example, the feeling that condom use will reduce enjoyment. Behavioural responses are expressions of *behavioural* intentions or overt verbal or non-verbal reactions towards the attitude object, for example the expressed intention to use condoms.

Attitude theories have been widely used in order to predict individual behaviour. Attitude is also a central concept in the field of change, for example in agricultural extension and health education. It is expected that a positive attitude towards behaviour, e.g. physical exercise, will stimulate a person to actually perform that behaviour. However, the correlation between attitudes and behaviour is often found to be weak. The first and best-known study to test the assumption that attitudes serve as behavioural dispositions is LaPiere's study of racial prejudice.

LaPiere (1934) was interested in finding out whether racial prejudice could be predicted by self-reported attitudes towards minorities. He travelled throughout the United States in the company of a young Chinese couple. Out of the 251 restaurants they visited, only one refused them entry. About six months later, LaPiere sent a questionnaire to the same restaurants in which he also asked whether or not they were willing to accept Chinese people. Of the 128 responses received, over 90 per cent were negative. Other researchers soon reported negative relations between attitudes and behaviour as well, raising doubts about the assumed strong relationship between attitudes and behaviour. It became necessary to consider possible explanations for these weak relations (for a comprehensive historical review, we refer to Ajzen & Fishbein, 1980). It was realised that thinking of behaviours as being determined exclusively by attitudes is a tremendous oversimplification. This led to new theories, in which attitudes are still considered to be an important, but not the only, predictor of behaviour.

3.5 Theory of planned behaviour

The most influential theory has been the theory of reasoned action (Fishbein & Ajzen, 1975), later expanded to the theory of planned behaviour (Ajzen, 1985; Ajzen & Madden, 1986). The authors' point of departure is that the best predictor of behaviour is a person's *intention* to perform (or not to perform) that behaviour. For example, to predict whether an individual will perform physical exercise, the simplest approach is to ask whether he or she intends to do so. It is important, however, to know the reasons underlying this intention. According to the theory, a person's intention is a function of three basic determinants. The first determinant is personal in nature, i.e. attitude towards the behaviour; the second reflects social influence, i.e. the subjective norm; and the third is related to the perceived difficulty of performing the behaviour, i.e. perceived behavioural control.

The personal factor, *attitude toward the behaviour,* reflects the person's judgement that performing the behaviour is good or bad. It is the person's positive or negative evaluation of performing the behaviour. People may differ in their attitudes towards physical exercise, some having favourable and some having unfavourable attitudes. Attitudes are a function of *behavioural beliefs (bb)*, i.e. beliefs about the consequences of performing the behaviour, and of the evaluations of those consequences, i.e. *outcome evaluations (e)*. Beliefs about performing physical exercise, for example, could be: it is likely that it will enhance my fitness, it will prevent me from getting fat, it will increase my cognitive capacity, improve my health, or perhaps, it will bring me interesting social contacts. Or they could be: it leads to injuries, it makes me tired, or it is time consuming. Each of these beliefs is connected with an evaluation (positive or negative; good or bad). The summed product of the behavioural beliefs and evaluations constitutes the attitude towards physical exercise (see Figure 3.4). Generally, a person who believes that performing a given behaviour will lead to mostly positive outcomes will hold a positive attitude towards performing that behaviour, whereas a person who believes that performing the behaviour will mostly lead to negative outcomes will hold a negative attitude. If we study attitudes in order to explain or predict behaviour, both behavioural beliefs and evaluation of these beliefs have to be measured at a high level of specificity. For instance, a general attitude towards healthy nutrition will only have a weak relationship with the choice to adopt a low-fat diet. To predict this behaviour, we have to measure the attitudes towards adopting a low-fat diet, thereby taking into account that a change in such behaviour usually has both favourable (e.g. lowers cholesterol levels, reduces weight) and unfavourable (less tasty, more expensive) consequences.

The second determinant of intention is the *subjective norm*. This is the perception of a person of the social pressures from 'important others' to perform or not to perform the behaviour in question. The person may feel that important others think he or she should - or should not - take up physical exercise. Subjective norms are a function of *normative beliefs (nb)*, i.e. the individual's belief that each of a number of significant others expects him or her to act in a certain way, and the *motivation to comply (mc)*, that is, the individual's inclination to live up to these others' expectations. Significant others may be parents, partner, siblings, peers, but also a doctor or a colleague. Generally, important others are those who are in control of positive and negative sanctions, i.e. those who can provide or withhold rewards. A person may believe that others think that he or she should or should not perform physical exercise. As with attitudes, each belief is multiplied by its corresponding motivation to comply. The sum of these products is the subjective norm (see Figure 3.4). The importance of others may depend on the type of behaviour or on the context. In the decision to wear protective gear at work, for example, the perceived expectation of colleagues may be more important than the perceived expectations of friends. For other kind of behaviours, friends or parents may be more important. The choice to adopt a low-fat diet may be highly influenced by the perceived expectations of the nearest family members (partner or children), whereas the perceived expectations of the doctor may only have a minor influence. For the measurement of subjective norms, we have to consider whose expectations regarding the specific behaviour are important, and what kinds of expectations the person thinks they hold regarding that behaviour.

Several studies have shown that attitudes and subjective norms are fair predictors of intention. If both are positive, the intention to perform a specific behaviour will be strong. The intention reduces if one or both are neutral or negative. However, it has often been found that attitudes and subjective norms only partially predict an individual's intention, and also the relation between intention and behaviour may be weak. To improve the predictive value of the theory, Ajzen (1985; 1988; 1991) expanded the model to the theory of planned behaviour, by adding the construct of *perceived behavioural control*. This construct represents the individual's perception of how easy or difficult it is to perform that specific behaviour. The construct is derived from Bandura's (1977; 1982) self-efficacy theory. According to Bandura, behaviour is a function of efficacy expectations and outcome expectations. *Outcome expectancy* is defined as a person's estimate that a given behaviour will lead to certain outcomes. Note that this concept compares to what we previously described as an attitude. *Efficacy expectation* is the conviction that one can successfully execute the behaviour required to produce the desired outcomes.

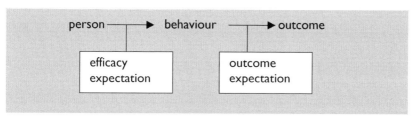

Figure 3.3 Representation of the difference between efficacy expectation and outcome expectation (Source: Bandura, 1977: 193).

Outcome and efficacy expectations are differentiated. Individuals can believe that a particular course of action will produce certain outcomes, but if they entertain serious doubts about whether *they are able to perform* the necessary activities, they will not take that course of action. The difference is presented schematically in Figure 3.3. So, individuals can believe that physical exercise will lead to improved fitness, but if they entertain serious doubts about whether they can perform the necessary activities, they will not perform physical exercise. Efficacy expectations determine how much effort people will expend and how long they will persist in the face of obstacles and aversive experiences. Self-efficacy therefore has motivational implications: if one believes one can succeed in a task, one is more likely to persist in the attempt despite early setbacks. The stronger the perceived self-efficacy is, the more active the efforts.

The concept of self-efficacy is similar to perceived behavioural control. Like attitudes and subjective norms, perceived behavioural control is based on beliefs, the so-called *control beliefs*. To assess perceived behavioural control it is helpful to consider Bandura's notions about the sources of efficacy expectations. These are performance accomplishments (experience, exposure), vicarious experience (live modelling, symbolic modelling), verbal persuasion (e.g. suggestion), and emotional arousal. Performance accomplishment has the strongest influence. In fact, it refers to the attribution of success or failure to internal or external causes, which we discussed earlier. Previous successful performances will lead to high levels of perceived behavioural control, whereas previous failures will lead to low levels of perceived behavioural control. Perceived behavioural control influences the intention to perform behaviour. A person with a high level of perceived control is more likely to act on that intention, including in the face of obstacles and setbacks, than a person who has a low level of perceived control. It should be noted that perceived behavioural control could also have a direct influence on behaviour. This is the case if individuals so strongly believe themselves to be unable to perform the behaviour that they do not even consider doing so.

The theory of planned behaviour is summarised in Figure 3.4. Attitudes, subjective norms and perceived behavioural control

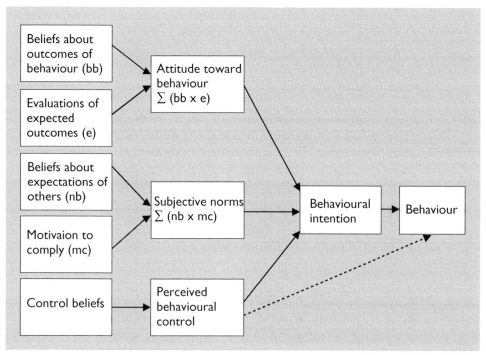

Figure 3.4 Theory of planned behaviour.

determine a person's intention to perform a certain behaviour. It should be realised, however, that individuals, given a positive intention, also must *be able* to perform the behaviour. This means that a person must have the necessary skills and there should be no major environmental constraints preventing behavioural performance (Fishbein & Yzer, 2003). Generally, the more favourable the attitude and subjective norm, and the greater the perceived behaviour control, the stronger is the person's intention to perform the behaviour in question. If a person additionally possesses the necessary skills and abilities to perform the behaviour, and if there are no environmental constraints on conducting the behaviour, there is a good chance that the behaviour will be performed.

3.5.1 Value of the theory

The theory of planned behaviour stems from the domain of cognitive social psychology. It has been applied in several fields, for example in marketing, environmental communication and agricultural extension, as well as within the domain of health behaviour. This includes, for example, programmes aiming to prevent children from taking up smoking, (*cf.* De Vries *et al.*, 1995; Leventhal & Cleary, 1980), or predicting and influencing adolescents' intentions to drink alcohol (e.g. Aas *et al.*, 1995; Oei *et al*, 1998), but it is also used in the field of nutrition (e.g. Vaandrager & Koelen, 1997), physical exercise (e.g. Biddle, 1992; Hausenblas *et al.*, 1998), and the prevention of HIV/AIDS (e.g. Schaalma, 1995). It should be noted that the measurement of attitudes can be rather time-consuming, due to the required specificity of that measurement, as we discussed previously. The theory, however, functions as a good device for understanding health behaviours, and therefore it gives clear indications for effective communicative interventions.

3.6 Theories on health behaviour

The attribution theory and the theory of planned behaviour are general theories, based in the domain of social psychology. Other theories have been developed specifically to address health-related behaviour. Here we elaborate on two models that try to explain why people do or do not engage in health protective behaviour: the health belief model (Janz & Becker, 1984) and the protection motivation theory (Rogers, 1975).

3.6.1 The health belief model

According to the health belief model (HBM; see Figure 3.5), health behaviour is determined by (1) belief in a personal health threat, and (2) belief in the effectiveness of a health behaviour. Belief in a personal health threat is effected firstly by the *perceived susceptibility* to a disease. This is the subjective risk of acquiring an illness if no countermeasures are taken, for example the estimated risk of acquiring cancer or HIV/AIDS. The second issue is the *perceived severity* of a disease. This is expressed in the perceived physical (e.g. pain, handicap, death) or social (e.g. infecting others, inability to work, economic difficulties) consequences of getting the disease. Perceived susceptibility and perceived severity determine the *belief in a personal health threat*. They invoke a general motivation for action. Individuals who feel threatened will look for ways to reduce the threat, that is, they

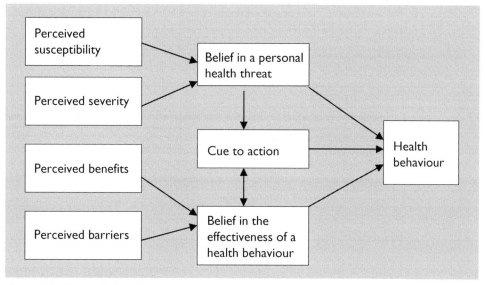

Figure 3.5 The health belief model.

will consider the performance of preventive behaviour. In fact, perceived susceptibility and perceived severity are the building blocks of fear. If both are at a high level, fear is also at a high level. If one of them is zero, there will be no fear. For example, the severity of HIV/AIDS may be clear. Yet, one person will experience high levels of fear, because of a high level of perceived vulnerability, whereas another person may not experience fear at all, because of a low level of perceived vulnerability.

Belief in the effectiveness of a health behaviour is a function of two beliefs; firstly, the perceived degree to which preventive behaviour will reduce the threat of the particular health risk. This is referred to as the *perceived benefits* of preventive behaviour. The second belief relates to the *perceived barriers*. These are the perceived negative aspects of a particular preventive behaviour, such as financial costs, social costs, and effort. Perceived benefits and perceived barriers determine the *belief in effectiveness* of a particular health measure to reduce risk, and this guides the choices for a particular behaviour.

Fundamental to the HBM is the existence of some form of awareness of a threat. This is called a *cue to action*, a precipitating force that makes the person feel the need to take action. Cues to action include a diverse range of triggers. They can be internal (e.g. individual perception of symptoms) or external (e.g. social influence or health education campaigns). For example, a 45-year-old man might feel that he runs the risk of getting cardiovascular disease. Contracting this disease clearly has severe consequences. He therefore might consider various alternative actions in order to reduce the risk, such as physical exercise, adopting a low-fat diet or stopping smoking. Each of these actions will reduce the risks, but also have some costs. For example, the man may believe that a low-fat diet is less tasty, or more expensive. According to the model, it is still possible that the man will take no action to reduce the risk until there is some cue to action. This could be an article in a newspaper indicating that men in their forties are particularly susceptible to the development of cardiovascular disease, or an annual health check up showing that his cholesterol level is too high. The model thus consists of six constructs. Yet, the relationships between the variables have never been spelled out or formalised (Stroebe & de Wit, 1996), and even the definition of the constructs has been left open to debate. Thus, even though one can question the status of the model as a coherent psychological model of prerequisites of health behaviour, the model allows the identification of beliefs correlated with health behaviours (*cf.* Janz & Becker, 1984).

3.6.2 Protection motivation theory

The protection motivation theory (Rogers, 1975; 1983) partially resembles the health belief model, but adds some interesting concepts. Whereas the HBM describes the factors that positively influence the motivation to health-enhancing behaviour, the protection motivation theory also describes forces that negatively influence this motivation. The theory begins with the notion that adaptive and maladaptive coping with a health threat is the result of two appraisal processes: (1) a process of *threat appraisal* and (2) a process of *coping appraisal* in which the behavioural options to diminish the threat are evaluated. The processes together result in either high or low protection motivation. High motivation produces the intention to perform adaptive responses; low motivation may lead to maladaptive responses, i.e. responses that place an individual in a health risk situation. The theory is illustrated in Figure 3.6. *Threat appraisal* is a function of two sets of beliefs, one inhibiting and the other facilitating health-impairing behaviour. The

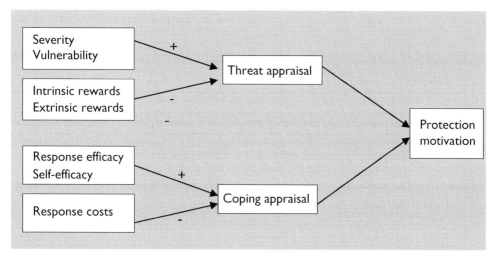

Figure 3.6 Protection motivation theory.

first set, similar to the 'belief in a personal health threat' in the HBM, consists of the *perceived severity* of the consequences of a disease, and the *perceived vulnerability* to (probability of) contracting the disease. Thus, perceived vulnerability and severity facilitate the probability of adaptive responses. The second set of beliefs consists of the potential rewards associated with the health-impairing behaviour. This is an important addition, since health-impairing behaviour most often involves some kind of reward. The rewards can be either intrinsic (e.g. the enjoyment of unprotected sex) or extrinsic (e.g. it is good for my image). Protection motivation is reduced if the potential intrinsic or extrinsic rewards of the health-impairing behaviour (e.g. enjoyment of unprotected sex) are high, and consequently it facilitates maladaptive behaviour.

The process of *coping appraisal* is also a function of two sets of beliefs, one inhibiting and the other facilitating health-impairing behaviour. The first set compares to the 'belief in the effectiveness of a health behaviour' in the HBM. It consists of *response efficacy*, i.e. the perceived effectiveness of the recommended behaviour in avoiding the negative consequences, and *self-efficacy*, i.e. the perceived ability to successfully execute the behaviour required to produce the outcomes. According to the theory, protection motivation is enhanced by the belief that the advised behaviour is effective in reducing the threat (e.g. using a condom prevents me from becoming infected with HIV), and by the expectation that one can successfully perform the advised behaviour (e.g. it is easy for me to use condoms). The second set of beliefs is again an important addition. It relates to *response costs*. A change in behaviour always involves some costs, for example, the loss of enjoyment associated with the risk behaviour. If the costs of the adaptive behaviour are perceived to be high (e.g. use of condoms reduces sexual enjoyment), this will limit protection motivation.

3.6.3 Value of the models

An important concept in both models is fear. Interventions to stimulate individuals to change health risk behaviours often use fear-arousing strategies. It is assumed that fear drives and motivates behaviour. Janis (1967) argues that the relation between the level of evoked fear and preparedness to follow the advised adaptive behaviour is parabolic. This implies that some level of fear is necessary to motivate a person to take action (see cue to action in the health belief model), a medium level of evoked fear leads to maximal adoption of the advised behaviour, and too high a level of fear leads to maladaptive responses, such as denial of the threat. Sutton (1982) conducted a meta-analysis on studies of the effects of fear on intentions and behaviour. He found that increases in fear are consistently associated with increases in intentional and behavioural measures of acceptance. Sutton did not find support for the parabolic function, that is, that excessively high levels of fear are counter-effective. However, even though there is no hard evidence, it is easy to think of practical examples in which the experience by people of high levels of fear leads to denial of the threat. Moreover, in the field of patient education it is known that people rarely comprehend information when they are emotionally upset (*cf.* DiMatteo & DiNicola, 1982). Consider, for example, a patient visiting a doctor to hear about the results of a cancer screening. Due to anxiety, patients become distracted from what is being said to them, and explanations will do little to change their state of knowledge about their condition unless their anxiety levels are reduced.

Another important contribution that can be derived from the models relates to the conditions influencing the change of health-impairing behaviour. In his meta-analysis, Sutton (1982) found that intentions to adopt healthier behaviour are influenced by the perceived efficacy of the recommended behaviour. Furthermore, providing specific instructions about how to perform the recommended behaviour leads to higher rates of acting in accordance with the recommendations. This implies that we should not focus merely on the negative consequences of the health-impairing behaviour. The costs and benefits (including intrinsic and extrinsic rewards) of both the existent behaviour and the advised behaviour need consideration. In addition, clear instructions about how to perform the alternative behaviour are essential.

The health belief model and the protection motivation theory have been applied and tested as to their usefulness in several studies relating to a variety of health-related topics. Three broad areas can be identified: (a) preventive health behaviours, which include health promotive (e.g. diet, exercise) and health risk behaviours (e.g. smoking, unsafe sex), as well as vaccination and contraceptive practices; (b) sick role behaviours, which refer to compliance with recommended medical regimes, usually following professional diagnosis of illness; and (c) clinic use, which includes physician visits for a variety of reasons (Sheeran & Abraham, 1996). Even though both models have strengths and weaknesses, and the assumed relations do not always appear to be strong in research, they contribute substantially to the understanding of the factors that determine the intention to perform certain behaviour.

3.7 Social influence

The theories described in the previous sections focus on the individual and individuals' cognitions. Some of these theories recognise the importance of the social environment - see for example the subjective norm, which refers to the indirect influence of important others - but individual information processing is seen to be the central drive in behaviour and behavioural change. Nevertheless, much behaviour, including health behaviour, occurs or is learnt in a social context. People spend a vast amount of time each day in groups of various sizes, for example family, schools, work places, sports clubs and churches. These groups exert influence on individual behaviour. Besides, it is clear that the attitudes of individuals are also strongly rooted in the groups to which people belong. Thus, if one wishes to understand human behaviour, it is necessary to take into account social influence as well.

We will now discuss how the social environment directly or indirectly influences attitudes and behaviour.

3.7.1 Normative and informational social influence

The study of social influence has a long tradition. In 1935, Sherif investigated the influence of social context on individual perception. In this experiment, three subjects sat in a completely darkened room, looking at a point of light waving back and forth in the distance. They were asked to judge how far the light moved. The light was actually physically stationary and only seemed to be moving. This illusion is called the 'auto kinetic effect'. The walls were not visible, and there were no other frames of reference for the subjects to use. Because the stimulus was so ambiguous, the first estimates of the three subjects differed considerably. After a while however, their estimates converged. They developed a common perception, a shared way of viewing the light. Next, each subject was alone in the darkened room, and again had to estimate how far the light moved. It appeared that these estimates were similar to the common perception as developed in the group. Thus, in this experiment the group defined an ambiguous stimulus in a certain way, and the individual then carried the group's definition with him when he was alone.

Other research on influence of the social context was conducted by Ash (1951; 1956). Ash had groups of eight subjects sit around a table. They were shown four lines, a standard line and three others of varying lengths (see Figure 3.7). Their task was to say which of the three lines was the same length as the standard line. Contrary to the task in Sherif's experiment, the subject could easily see which was right. The experiment began with each subject expressing his judgement aloud. However, only one out of the eight subjects (number 6) was a real subject. The others were confederates of the experimenter. After some trials in which each gave the right answer, suddenly the confederates gave an answer that was clearly wrong. In these situations, 40 per cent of the subjects gave the wrong answer as well, even though they knew that the answer was wrong.

The studies of both Sherif and Ash demonstrate social influence: the individual responses were influenced by the responses of the others. There is a difference, however, in the type of social influence. The influence in the Sherif study is called informational social influence.

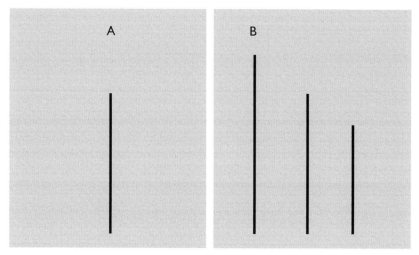

Figure 3.7 Representative stimulus in the Ash's study.

The subjects had to perform an ambiguous task and had no reference for the right or wrong answer. They therefore used each other's judgements as information for their own estimation. The influence in the Ash studies is called normative social influence. The importance of differentiating between these two types of social influence relates to the impact on the individual. The convergence of individuals' thoughts, feelings and behaviour towards a group norm is called *conformity*. The impact of normative social influence, however, is usually restricted to the specific situation in which the norm is important. In another context, the impact disappears. This is called *public conformity* or *compliance*. Ash demonstrated this effect when he asked the 'real subjects', after the group session, to judge the lines once again. All of them then gave the correct answers. However, when people are truly persuaded that the group is right, and when they accept the group norms as their own beliefs, *private conformity* or *acceptance* occurs. The impact of informational social influence is long lasting. This means not only that a person alters his or her opinion, attitude or behaviour as long as he or she is in the specific context, but also that the information from the group is indeed accepted and internalised. This is what happened in the Sherif experiment also: the individual carried the group's definition with him when he was alone. So, informational social influence can convince a person. It leads to acceptation of the group norm and has a longer lasting impact.

Normative social influence leads to adaptation to the norm, only for as long as one is in the specific context.

3.7.2 Norms

An essential element in social influence is what we call 'social norms'. Social norms can be considered as a set of values that define the range of acceptable and unacceptable attitudes and behaviours for members of a social unit. Norms specify certain rules or ways in which group members should behave. As such, they are the basis for mutual expectations among the group members. A norm can apply to a society (general norms), but also to communities (e.g. geographical areas, school or workplace), or smaller groups, such as a family or a group of friends (group norms). For individuals, norms act as a frame of reference. Norms can bring order and predictability, especially to ambiguous situations. This is exactly what happened in the Sherif study previously described. When objective criteria are unavailable, social groups are inclined to formulate their own 'rights' and 'wrongs'. Norms regulate the existence and co-ordination of groups. In everyday life, individuals show consistency in their behaviour and in their expression of, for example, attitudes and opinions. Inconsistency would make organised social interaction difficult. Acting consistently, according to established norms, results in predictability and regularity in behaviour and creates stability in social relations. In studies on social influence, we found that individuals who comply with this so-called consistency norm receive social approval and acceptance, whereas individuals acting inconsistently elicit negative feelings in others. Violation of norms by a group member will lead to pressure from other group members to 'correct' the deviant. If these influence attempts are unsuccessful, the group members come to dislike the deviant and ultimately expel him or her from the group. Norms are influential for all kinds of behaviour, including health-related behaviour. Many health-related behaviours, such as smoking, alcohol and food consumption, have a social function and are subject to mutual expectations of those involved in these social situations. In a study on adolescent smoking behaviour (Koelen, 1988), we found that smokers and non-smokers showed significant differences not only in the number of their friends who smoked, but also in the behaviours and activities they engaged in (e.g. going to a bar or disco, practising sports), as well as in their preference for a particular style of clothing. On the other hand, we found a surprisingly strong correlation between the ways in which adolescents act and their peers' expectations: smokers and non-smokers were equally eager to meet the expectations of their friends on a wide range of behaviours, including how they interacted with each other. This is particularly interesting since both categories value different behaviours and activities.

Health-related behaviour is not an isolated form of behaviour; it takes place in a social context. Behaviours are embedded in social relationships and in the habits of the group (or groups) to which a person belongs. Consequently, social influence is an important determinant of individual behaviour. Social influence is a two-way influence, in that it is rewarding for both the individual and group to live up to each other's expectations. These expectations can either stimulate or prevent unhealthy behaviour. In attempting to change or maintain health-related behaviour, we therefore have to take into account the social environment in which those behaviours occur.

3.8 Chapter summary

In this chapter we have described theories that are important for understanding health behaviour and the processes underlying behavioural change. Firstly we described the ways in which people receive stimuli, and factors influencing the interpretation of those stimuli. Next we discussed attribution theories, explaining that people are not mere perceivers, but that they actively try to *explain* and *understand* the things they perceive. We then continued with the concepts of attitudes, subjective norms, self-efficacy, fear and social influence and the function of these concepts in understanding behaviour and behaviour change. It is clear that these theories can be helpful in analysing health-related behaviour, and in finding possibilities to induce behavioural change. It is not easy to say which theory is the most helpful. This will depend on the type of behaviour on which we are focusing, the complexity of this behaviour, and the (social) function of the behaviour in the wider context of lifestyles.

4. Individual and collective change

Health education and health promotion programmes are designed to stimulate individuals and groups to maintain healthy behaviours, to change unhealthy ones, or to adopt new behaviours conducive to health. For example, we encourage people to change dietary habits, to consume less alcohol, or to practice safe sex. In the previous chapter we presented and discussed theories that help us to understand and predict health-related behaviour. This chapter focuses on theories and models describing *processes of change,* at both the individual and the social level. Firstly, in section 4.1, we present two models that describe the stages an individual has to go through in the process of behavioural change. In 4.2 our focus is on collective change.

4.1 Individual change

Usually, behaviour change involves replacing existing behaviour with 'new behaviour', and therefore relates to the adoption of innovations. According to Rogers (1995:11), an innovation is ' ... an idea, practice, or object perceived as new by an individual. It matters little, so far as human behaviour is concerned, whether or not an idea is "objectively" new as measured by the lapse of time since its first discovery. It is the perceived (subjective) newness of the idea that determines people's reaction to it. If the idea seems new to the individual, it is an innovation'. The metric system, for example, is still an innovation for some Anglo Saxon people, despite the fact that it was developed over 200 years ago. But what decision-making pathways do individuals follow when considering whether or not to adopt an innovation? In his book *Diffusion of innovations,* Rogers (1995) proposes five different stages in this so-called adoption process: knowledge, persuasion (forming and changing attitudes), decision (adoption or rejection), implementation, and confirmation. The model of adoption processes originates from studies in the field of agriculture, but has been adapted for use in other areas too, including the specific field of health. Two of these models are presented here: the precaution adoption process model, and the transtheoretical model of behaviour change.

4.1.1 The precaution adoption process model

The precaution adoption process model (Weinstein, 1988) combines the abovementioned adoption process with concepts of the health belief model and protection motivation theory (see section 3.6). The model is illustrated in Figure 4.1.

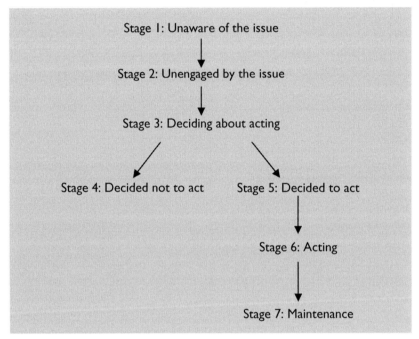

Figure 4.1 Stages of the precaution adoption process model.

The model begins with the individual who is unaware of a given health risk (stage 1), either because the risk is as yet generally unknown (e.g. before 1980, the risk of HIV infection; before 1995, the risk of RSI from working on a computer everyday) or out of personal ignorance. When individuals first learn about a certain health risk, they are no longer unaware, but they still may not be concerned by this knowledge (stage 2). Consider the example we used in Chapter 3 of the 45-year-old man who is aware of the risks of high cholesterol levels but does not take action to reduce the risk until there is some cue to action. This could be an article in a newspaper indicating that men, especially those in their forties, are particularly susceptible to the development of cardiovascular disease, or perhaps an annual health check, showing that his cholesterol level is too high. This so-called 'cue to action' would move him to stage 3, the stage at which decisions are being considered. The decision can be either not to take action (stage 4) or to take action (stage 5). If the person decides not to take action, the precaution adoption process stops, at least at this particular point in time. If the person decides to act however, the next step is to actually initiate action (stage 6). In our example, the man may decide to see a dietician in order to go on a low cholesterol diet. If the person continues the new behaviour, he will arrive at the stage of maintenance (stage 7). Note that stage 7 is essential as far as repetitive behaviour is concerned. If a person decides to stop smoking (stage 5) and implements this decision today (stage 6) but lights up a cigarette first thing the next morning, it will not be very effective. The same holds true for behaviours like physical exercise, food intake, safe sex or alcohol consumption. Stage 7 is not important when single actions are required, for example in the case of polio vaccination.

4.1.2 The transtheoretical model of behaviour change

The transtheoretical model of behaviour change distinguishes five stages of change through which individuals move when changing their behaviour, that is: precontemplation, contemplation, preparation, action, and maintenance. Although the terminology differs from the adoption process model, the contents of the stages are comparable. An advantage of the transtheoretical model is that it pays explicit attention to the *processes of change* in each stage, and therefore it helps us to understand when particular shifts in attitudes, intentions and behaviour occur, and how these shifts occur. The model postulates that behaviour change is not a dichotomous event, but a multi-step cyclical process through one or more of the distinct stages. In the description of the model we follow the work of the founders (Prochaska *et al.*, 1992).

The stages of change
Precontemplation is the stage in which individuals have no intention to change behaviour in the foreseeable future (in terms of the theory: the next six months). This stage includes individuals who are unaware of the problem behaviour and have not thought about the desirability of changing behaviour; those who have thought about it, but arrived at

the conclusion that they do not need or do not wish to change; and those who are demoralised by unsuccessful previous change attempts. Resistance to recognising or modifying a problem is the hallmark of precontemplation. Individuals in the *contemplation* stage are aware that a problem exists as well as of the need for behaviour change. This means that there is a gap between the existing and the desired situation. In this stage, individuals are seriously thinking about taking action, but have not yet made a commitment to actually start changing. A person in this stage may feel some unease about the impact of his or her health-impairing behaviour, but still will not have taken the decision to change. Individuals actively weigh up the advantages (pros) and disadvantages (cons) of the existing behaviour and the new behaviour. They can remain in this stage for a long period of time. Individuals in this stage will indicate that they are seriously considering changing their behaviour in the near future (according to the theory: within the next six months). Individuals in the *preparation stage* have formed the intention to take action in the immediate future, usually measured as the next month. They often have a plan of action and will report some small behaviour changes, but have not yet reached the criterion for effective action as agreed upon by scientists and professionals to be sufficient to reduce risks for diseases. For example, a person who has formed the intention to adopt a low cholesterol diet has already begun to stop using butter with breakfast, but continues to eat all other foods. *Action* is the stage in which individuals make specific modifications in their lifestyle in order to overcome their problems. Action involves overt behavioural changes and requires considerable commitment of time and energy on the part of the individual. People are classified as being in this stage if they have actually and successfully altered their behaviour (e.g. adopted a recommended diet) for a period of time, ranging from one day to six months. *Maintenance* is the stage in which individuals make a great effort to prevent relapse and to consolidate. According to Prochaska *et al.* (1992), this stage begins six months after the initial action and continues for an indeterminate period. For some behaviours, maintenance can be considered to last a lifetime. Being able to consistently engage in a new behaviour for more than six months is a criterion for considering someone to be in the maintenance stage.

Originally, Prochaska *et al.* (1992) considered behaviour change as a linear process. This would mean that, as soon as a person reached the stage of action, the health-impairing behaviour would definitely be modified into health-conducive behaviour. However, the numbers of people that relapse to the previous behaviour quite often outnumber those that persist in the newly adopted behaviour. In studies on, for example, smoking or dietary behaviour, relapse percentages often reach 60 to 80 per cent or more, and quite often people make an average of three to four action attempts before they become long-term maintainers. Since relapse is the rule rather than the exception, Prochaska and Velicer (1997) changed the original linear conception to assume a spiral pattern, in which people can progress from contemplation to preparation to action to maintenance, although most individuals will relapse. During relapse, individuals regress to an earlier stage. Some relapsers feel like failures, become demoralised and resist thinking about behaviour change. They return to the precontemplation stage and can remain there for varying periods of time. Others, however, return to the contemplation or preparation stages. They begin to consider plans for their next action attempt whilst trying to learn from their recent efforts. Whether they are motivated to take new action also depends on whether they attribute their relapse to, for example, stable (ability) or unstable (effort) causes (see section 3.3).

Processes of change
The stages of change are intertwined with processes of change, and this enables us to understand *how* the shift between stages occurs. These processes reflect the cognitive and behavioural techniques employed by individuals to alter certain behaviour. Ten processes throughout the stages of change were supported through research (*cf.* Rossi *et al.*, 1994; Prochaska & Velicer, 1997; Horwath, 1999). The strategies can be distinguished in two broad categories. The first category consists of experiential or cognitive processes, and includes activities relating to thinking and experiencing emotions about changing behaviour:
1. consciousness raising: becoming aware of the causes, consequences and solutions for the problem behaviour, for example by means of observations and confrontations;
2. dramatic relief: experiencing and expressing emotions, feelings of unease, and the motivation to reduce negative feelings through adequate action;
3. environmental re-evaluation: assessing the impact of the problem behaviour on the physical and social environment;
4. self-revaluation: assessing how one feels about oneself with respect to the problem behaviour;

5. self-liberation: choosing and commitment to act, or belief in one's own capabilities to modify the behaviour.

The second category consists of behavioural processes that are assumed to be helpful for changing the behaviour:

6. reinforcement management: managing the consequences of the behaviour in terms of positive and negative sanctioning;
7. helping relationships: a combination of care, trust, acceptance and support of others in changing the behaviour;
8. counter-conditioning: learning to substitute alternatives for the problem behaviour, replacing the existing behaviour with the new behaviour;
9. stimulus control: removal or avoidance of stimuli that elicit problem behaviours;
10. social liberation: an increase in numbers of alternatives for non-problem behaviours available.

It is assumed that the processes in the first category are of special relevance in the stages of precontemplation, contemplation and preparation, whereas the processes in the second category are important in the stages of action and maintenance.

4.1.3 Relation to determinants of behaviour

The stages and processes of change can be related to several of the determinants of behaviour as described in Chapter 3. In the stage of precontemplation in particular, attitudes and the perceptions of severity and vulnerability are important. In the contemplation stage, the individual actively weighs up the pros and cons. This indeed forms the basis for a positive or negative attitude towards the behaviour. In the preparation, action and maintenance stage, perceived self-efficacy is important. In the action and maintenance stage, the (perceived) expectations and the actual support or disapproval of others either help or hinder the individual in persisting with the new behaviour (*cf.* Amick & Ockene, 1994; Verheijden *et al.*, 2003). Hence subjective norms and direct social influence play an important role, especially in the later stages. The relationship between stages, processes and determinants is illustrated in Table 4.1.

Table 4.1 Overview of stages of change and the cognitive and behavioural processes.

Stages	Processes	Determinants
Precontemplation	1. Consciousness raising	Awareness
	2. Dramatic relief	Attitudes
	3. Environmental re-evaluation	Severity / vulnerability
Contemplation	4. Self-evaluation	
Preparation	5. Self liberation	
Action	6. Reinforcement management	Self-efficacy
	7. Helping relations	Subjective norms
	8. Counter conditioning	Social influence
	9. Stimulus control	
Maintenance	10. Social liberation	

4.1.4 Implications of the stage models

Professionals frequently carefully design interventions aimed to influence certain health-related behaviour, but the number of people actually modifying their behaviour often disappoints them. One of the advantages of the transtheoretical model is that it focuses on the change *process*. In addition, it emphasises that interventions have to be adapted to the stage of change of the target individuals, rather than assuming one intervention will be equally applicable to all. This is also referred to as *tailoring*, that is: 'any combination of information or change strategies intended to reach one specific person, based on characteristics that are unique to that person, related to the outcome of interest, and have been derived from an individual assessment' (Kreuter *et al.*, 2000:5). The transtheoretical model thus provides a methodological approach to characterising people's awareness of, and readiness to, adopt health behaviour. People are unlikely to do anything about a health problem unless they are aware of its existence. Information about the health consequences of health-impairing behaviour is therefore needed for those in the precontemplation or contemplation stage. This information has to aim at increasing awareness of the problem and has to address the individual's attitudes towards the existing and the new behaviour. It enables the individual to weigh up the pros and cons and to take a decision to act. Once the decision to act has been taken, action and maintenance-oriented information, for example information that enhances the self-efficacy of the individual with regard to changing the behaviour, is more effective (Stroebe, 2000). In addition, practical advice and instruction to learn both to adopt the new behaviour and to avoid or cope with stimuli that elicit the health-impairing behaviour are essential in these stages. It is clear that especially in these stages involvement of the social context (including indirect and direct social influences) in which the behaviour occurs is important. Thus, matching the information and support given to individuals to the stage of change is a way to optimise the effectiveness of any intervention. Specific guidelines for the design of successful interventions can be derived from the theoretical models as described in Chapter 3. Although research results do not always support the theoretical assumptions underlying the stage models (*cf.* Stroebe, 2000), there is evidence that tailored-to-stage interventions are more effective than interventions that disregard the stages or aim at the 'wrong' stages (Kreuter & Skinner, 2000). Ockene *et al.* (1988), for example, found that an intensive action- and maintenance-oriented smoking cessation programme for cardiac patients was highly successful for patients in the action stage, but unsuccessful for smokers in the precontemplation and contemplation stages. Similar results have been found in the fields of nutrition, weight control, physical activity, the use of mammography services, and screening behaviour for colorectal cancer (*cf.* Rakowski, 1992; Ashworth, 1997; Steptoe *et al.*, 2001; Verheijden *et al.*, 2003; Trauth *et al.*, 2003).

4.2 Collective change

The theories and models described so far focus on understanding and predicting behaviour and behavioural change at the level of individuals. Health promotion, however, is fundamentally directed towards improving the health of populations, and not merely the health of individuals. As discussed in section 2.3, the Ottawa Charter on Health Promotion (WHO, 1986) explicitly emphasises the importance of concrete and effective community action in setting priorities for health, making decisions, planning strategies and implementing them to achieve better health. Therefore, the capacity of individuals to act collectively on issues affecting their health and the health of the communities to which they belong is important too. Although many individuals together add up to a collective, social change processes are more than the sum of a number of individual changes. A helpful approach towards the understanding of social change processes can be found in the diffusion of innovations theory, which we will describe in more detail.

4.2.1 Diffusion of innovations

Changes in groups, either small or large, do not occur overnight. Equally, not all members of a group will change at the same moment in time. Some people accept new ideas (innovations) very quickly, whereas others tend to be more suspicious of such innovations. Consider the spread of mobile phones in the 1990s, or the use of the Internet. In his diffusion of innovations theory, Rogers (1995) describes how diffusion of innovations proceeds. *Diffusion* is defined as *the process by which an innovation is communicated through certain channels over time among members of a social system.* More than 4,000 research reports have been published about the communication process involved in the diffusion or spread of innovations, and about how people decide whether to adopt or reject these innovations. Much of the research was carried out in US agriculture around 1950 because administrators were concerned about the delays in farmers' use of research findings. There was a boom in this research in less industrialised countries during the 1960s because ministries of agriculture saw the need for large numbers of farmers to use the results of scientific agriculture in order to prevent famine. In recent decades, many of these studies have been conducted in developing countries such as India, but they have also been carried out by market researchers in industrial countries (see Engel *et al.*, 1986:Ch.20). All this research was undertaken because people wanted to know how the adoption of relevant innovations could be accelerated. The research centred around five questions:

1. Which decision-making pathways do individuals follow when considering whether or not to adopt an innovation?
2. What are the differences between people who adopt innovations quickly and those who adopt them slowly (adopter categories)?
3. How do characteristics of innovations affect the rate of adoption?
4. How do potential users communicate amongst themselves about these innovations?
5. How does an innovation diffuse through society over time?

The first question focuses on the individual and has been addressed in the previous section. In the following section, the results of questions 2 - 5 will be discussed in more detail.

4.2.2 Adopter categories

Differences between people who readily adopt innovations and those who play a waiting game are an interesting topic for investigation. Rogers (1995) uses a system of classifying different adopters into five categories according to the time it takes for adoption to occur. These are:

1. *Innovators,* who are those 2.5 per cent of a population who are quickest to adopt new ideas. They are very eager to try new ideas. They actively seek information about new ideas, have a high degree of media exposure, and their interpersonal networks extend over a wide area, usually reaching beyond their local environment. Innovators are not always respected or trusted by other members of their social network. The role of the innovator in the diffusion process is that of launching new ideas into a social system.

2. *Early adopters* (13.5 per cent) are more integrated into the local social system than the innovators. This category has the greatest degree of opinion leadership in the community. They have some personal, social or financial resources to adopt the innovation, but they are not too far above average in terms of innovatory skills. The early adopter is respected by peers and is considered by many as the person to check with before using a new idea. The role of the early adopter is to decrease uncertainty about a new idea by adopting it, thereby providing a subjective evaluation for near-peers by means of interpersonal networks.

3. The *early majority* (34.0 per cent) is that part of the social system that adopts new ideas just before the average member of the system. They are persuaded by the benefits of adopting the innovation. In general, they interact frequently with their peers, but seldom have a leadership position. The early majority forms the important link between the very early and relativly late to adopt.

4. The *late majority* (34.0 per cent) is generally sceptical and cautious toward innovations, and people in this category do not adopt until most others in their social system have done so. Usually, pressure from peers is necessary to motivate adoption, and almost all of the uncertainty about the new idea has to be removed.

5. *Laggards* (16.0 per cent) are the last in a social system to adopt an innovation. In many cases they are suspicious and actively resistant to innovations. Most often they are rather isolated in a social system.

Classification of people in these different adopter categories by definition depends on the degree to which the whole group has adopted the innovations. Rogers suggests a normal, bell-shaped, distribution over time on a frequency basis as can be derived from the percentages for each category. The cummulative number of adopters results in an s-shaped curve. This is shown in Figure 4.2.

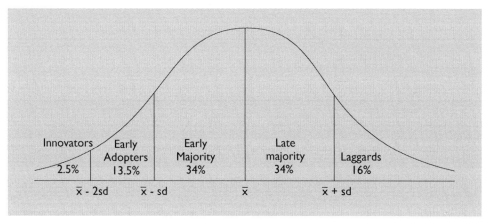

Figure 4.2 Adopter categorisation on the basis of innovativeness.

In several studies, the relationship between an individual's adoption index and a variety of his or her social characteristics have been investigated in such diverse areas as agriculture in industrialised and less industrialised countries, education, health services, and consumer behaviour. Remarkably similar results have been found in all of these fields. It appears to make little difference whether you are an American doctor or an Indian farmer. Some of the results are summarised in Table 4.2.

Care should be taken in interpreting this table because it does not distinguish between cause and effect. Many studies clearly show that people who have adopted many innovations have frequent contact with change agents. Is that because this contact results in the adoption of

Table 4.2 Percentage of studies showing positive relationships between adoption index and other variables.

Variable	% of studies in which positive relationship has been found	Number of research studies
Education	74	275
Literacy	63	38
Higher social status	68	402
Larger size units	67	227
Commercial economic orientation	71	28
More favourable attitude to credit	76	25
More favourable attitude to change	75	57
More favourable attitude to education	81	31
Intelligence	100	5
Social participation	73	149
Cosmopolitanism (urban contacts)	76	174
Change agent contact	87	156
Mass media exposure	69	116
Exposure to interpersonal channels	77	60
More active information seeking	86	14
Knowledge of innovations	76	55
Opinion leadership	76	55

Based on: Rogers, E.M. (1983) Diffusion of Innovations, 3rd edn., pp. 260-261. Free Press, New York.

innovations, because people interested in innovation seek contact with change agents, or because change agents seek contact with these people? Probably all three factors play some role. Also, some of the relationships, while positive, are very weak. Age is not included in Table 4.1 because, contrary to popular opinion, no relationship was found in about half of the studies, and only one third of the other studies showed that younger people are more innovative than older people.

Moreover, in interpreting these research findings we have to keep in mind that this kind of research has been undertaken for innovations which are considered to be useful for all members of a social system.

In reality, there are all sorts of innovations that are useful for some people but not for others, perhaps because they have different goals or aspirations. A private plane may be very useful to solve the transport problems of a rich businessman, but, for most people, a good bicycle is more useful. In addition, innovations may be very useful for large groups, but people may lack the necessary resources to adopt those innovations. For example, there are medicines that enable HIV/AIDS patients to live much longer, but they are out-of-reach for most of these patients because they cost many times their annual income (Singhal & Rogers, 2003). Besides, many innovations in health are not available to a large proportion of the population in developing countries, due to the poor organisation of the health care system. In studying adoption of innovations processes, it is important to analyse carefully whether people have good reasons not to adopt innovations recommended by an expert who, as a specialist, may focus his attention only on certain aspects of the problem.

Notwithstanding all that, investigations on diffusion of innovations allow us to predict the type of people who will quickly apply innovations in practice and the type who will not. It also shows that different innovations may take different time periods to introduce to the majority, and we have to realise that it takes time to reach an entire population, if they are reached at all. As Nutbeam and Harris (1998:41) argue, the increasing difficulty of influencing late adopters and laggards translates into diminishing returns on efforts in health programmes and needs to be recognised in the planning and evaluation of programmes.

The adopter categories differ in the extent to which they are integrated into the local social system. The early adopters, and the early majority in particular, are integrated into their communities and frequently interact with their peers. This indicates the importance of networks in communities, of communication channels, and something known as cohesion. Cohesion may be defined as 'the powers within a social system that are keeping the individuals inside that system'. Cohesion consists of the components 'neighbouring' and 'sense of community'. 'Neighbouring' refers to interaction between community members (e.g. talking to each other, paying visits), and to social support. 'Sense of community' includes four elements: identification and sense of belonging (personal relatedness), influence (a sense of making a difference to a group), shared emotional connection (the committment and belief that members have a shared history, common places of interest and similar experiences), and pressure to conform (McMillan & Chavis, 1986). The amount of cohesion in a social system influences the diffusion of information. The more cohesion, the quicker the circulation of information. Chavis and Wandersman (1990) show that sense of community functions as a catalyst for action. It has a positive influence on a person's perception of the environment, on social relations, and on the degree to which people become involved in matters affecting the social system. In a community project on nutrition promotion, it was found that, in neighbourhoods with strong community networks, residents participated far more actively in the project than in less cohesive neighbourhoods (Vaandrager, 1995; Koelen, 2000). Ecklund (1999) found similar results.

4.2.3 Characteristics of innovations

The rate of adoption, that is the relative speed by which an innovation is adopted by members of a social system, differs from innovation to innovation. Some innovations are adopted very quickly (for example, new fashions) whereas others require remarkably long periods of time. Rate of adoption can be partially explained by the perceived attributes of the innovation. Five characteristics that are consistently associated with successful adoption are:

- *Relative advantage* - i.e. the degree to which an innovation is perceived as better than the idea it supersedes. The degree of advantage can be expressed in terms of economic profitability or in social benefits like increased status or social approval, as well as decrease in discomfort, a saving of time and effort and immediacy of the reward. According to Rogers, this latter aspect explains in part why preventive innovations have an especially low rate of adoption. Generally, it is difficult to demonstrate the advantage of such innovations. The advantages of smoking, alcohol consumption and food consumption are typically immediate, whereas the advantage of changing these behaviours, i.e. a change in the probability of getting a disease, occurs somewhere in the unknown future.
- *Compatibility* is the degree to which an innovation is consistent with socio-cultural values and beliefs, needs, or with past experience. The use of contraceptives, for example, may be incompatible with some religious values.

- *Complexity* is the degree to which an innovation is perceived as difficult to understand or difficult to use. Innovations that require simple actions are more likely to be successful - for example, preparing healthier meals using the usual equipment and ingredients.
- *Trialability* refers to the extent to which an innovation may be tried out on a small scale. For example, a dietician who has to develop evidence-based methods of working might first want to try to work according to this new method on a small scale, before applying it to all clients. Similarly, someone may want to try out some sports first before paying a sports club for a year's membership. Triable innovations are less risky, and therefore more easily adopted.
- *Observability* refers to the degree to which the results of an innovation are visible to others. If someone observes a friend losing weight by following a diet, it may have an impact on that person's own decision to do so. This very much compares to Bandura's idea of modelling and vicarious learning (Bandura, 1986) we discussed in section 3.2.2. It should be noted that observability is also a difficult issue in preventive innovations (see relative advantage above).

We should realise that, generally, innovations do not meet *all* these criteria, but an understanding of these characteristics is important in designing health education and health promotion programmes. For example, when trying to convince cyclists to wear a helmet, we may easily find arguments about relative advantage. To use a helmet may not seem to be complicated, but are helmets available at easy-to-reach purchase points? (complexity). Trialability may be difficult too, because a helmet has to be bought. The example shows that consideration of these characteristics can also help to identify implementation problems.

4.2.4 The diffusion processes

How innovations diffuse through groups over time depends on how potential users communicate about the innovations. Previously, we mentioned that adoption of innovations is influenced strongly by members of social groups. Generally, when some members of a group have adopted an innovation, others will often follow. This relation is not always that straightforward however. The question is how we can influence the diffusion process within social groups.

Opinion leaders have considerable influence on the way in which people think and act. As it is impossible for health workers or other professionals to work closely with all members of a group or a larger community, it will be helpful to identify those members of the system who are considered to be opinion leaders. When we described adoption categories, we mentioned that opinion leaders are often found among the early adopters. Opinion leaders fulfil several of the following functions in their group or community with regard to innovations:

- passing on information from outside the group;
- interpreting this outside information on the basis of his or her own opinions and experience;
- setting an example for others to follow;
- 'legitimising' or rejecting changes that others want to carry out. That is, the opinion leader gives his or her approval or disapproval for these changes; and
- they are influential in changing group norms.

Usually, not all these functions are combined in one person. There may be some opinion leaders who provide information early in the adoption process and others who legitimise the decision to adopt or reject an innovation. In addition, we should take into account the meaning of 'community'. Community, community action and community participation are at the heart of health promotion, but there is no agreement about what a community actually is (we elaborate on this topic in section 7.1). We may see a certain geographical area as a community, but people living in those areas may not consider themselves to be members of the same community. Practically, according to Laverack and Labonte (2000), a community is best considered to be an organised group that is important enough to its individual members in that they identify themselves, in part, by that group membership. This implies that, within any geographic community, multiple communities actually exist and that each individual may belong to several different communities at the same time (Laverack & Labonte, 2000:258). Each of these different groups can have its own opinion leaders who have limited influence on other groups. The change agent may therefore have to look for opinion leaders in each of these groups. Because accepted community members can function as role models, they can help accelerate the rate of adoption.

Many innovations can only diffuse effectively among people who are more or less homogenous in, for example, resources, social status or religion. Some innovations that are suitable for one group are unsuitable for another group, especially where there are large differences in, for example, age, interests or lifestyle (see differences between smoking and non-smoking youngsters as reported in section 3.7.2). Social interaction between these groups is often limited. Moreover, in many cultures there are separate communication networks for men and women. In such cases, information given to male opinion leaders will often reach women very slowly, and, if it reaches them at all, the information is perhaps rather distorted. Change agents in these situations should try to establish contacts with opinion leaders from each of the groups.

4.3 Lessons for health education and health promotion

In section 4.1.2 we pointed out that the process of individual change is not a linear but rather an iterative process. Community change is also an iterative process. Rogers' theory helps us to explain how changes in communities can be facilitated. It stresses the importance of identifying opinion leaders and getting them involved in health promotion programmes at a very early stage. Opinion leaders usually belong to the category of early adopters and are well regarded by other community members. As such, they can function as role models, and they provide evaluation information about the innovation. Opinion leaders can be considered as peers in the respect that they have similar attributes to those with whom they communicate. They are different in some aspects too, in that they tend to have a slightly higher status, as well as being more educated and more innovative. Studies have shown that the involvement of community leaders is essential to programme success (*cf.* Bracht *et al.*, 1999).

Diffusion of innovations theory also emphasises that the spread of innovations takes time. Even if the benefits of an innovation seem to be obvious, it may diffuse at a very slow rate, and some innovations fail to get diffused at all. In this regard, Rogers (1995:10) mentions the Dvorak keyboard for typewriters that has several advantages over the Qwerty keyboard, but never quite made it. Additionally, for innovations that appear to diffuse at a fast rate in the first instance, it can take a very long time before the late majority will follow. As Tones and Tilford (1994:85) argue, it is clearly wise not to expect instant success, and health professionals have to take account of the fact that it will be increasingly difficult to influence later adopters as well as the residual hard core within the category of laggards. This also means that less ambitious standards have to be set when a programme is seeking to influence the late majority.

Diffusion theory is not only applicable to the introduction of new ideas (including the idea of community participation in health promotion) into communities. It can also be considered in relation to the involvement of organisations in health promotion, with special reference to intersectoral collaboration. This is of great importance, in terms of both creating supportive environments and the sustainability of programmes. Health promotion projects do not usually begin as a collective effort by many organisations. On the contrary, they arise mostly as a small project guided by only a few interested and motivated individuals and organisations. Indeed: the innovators. When these efforts are carried out sensitively and results become visible, early adopters will follow, etcetera. In a community-based nutrition promotion programme carried out in seven European (healthy) cities and that began in each city as a small project, it was found that particularly communication about the programme, the visibility of activities and its outcomes, and the visibility of the participants' contribution had an increasing spin-off in terms of participating organisations (Koelen, 2000). Examples of successes (success breeds success) are important in terms of both getting health issues onto the political agenda and convincing organisations to participate.

4.4 Chapter summary

The processes by which many types of innovations are adopted by individuals and the processes by which innovations diffuse have been studied extensively. Many years may pass between the time people first hear about some innovations and the time they adopt them. At community level, opinion leaders play an important role in diffusing innovations. They tend to be people who are capable, willing and in a position to help others solve important problems. Who becomes an opinion leader in a group depends on group norms and current problems facing the group. Messages about innovations will be most successful when the receiver trusts the source and shares similar attitudes towards the innovation. The ideas underlying diffusion theory are applicable not only at the level of individuals or communities, but also at the level of organisations. The rate of adoption is influenced by the perception of the characteristics of the innovation. Results of adoption research can be used to accelerate the rate of adoption of innovations or to change adoption processes in such a way that certain categories adopt innovations more rapidly. Hence, it may be necessary to develop different strategies for different categories.

5. Communication

Communication is essential not only in informing people about health concerns, but also in maintaining important health issues on the agenda. Simply stated, communication is the process that takes place if people or groups interact with each other. We communicate everyday, and for as long as we can remember. It is so much an integral part of life that usually we do not consciously think about it. Yet communication is a complex process, and there are several interrelated elements involved that influence the results of this process. In this chapter we review some fundamental aspects of communication, and we develop a model of the communication process. We go on to discuss important elements that affect the outcomes of communication processes and conclude by elaborating to some extent on the influence of selective perception. Selective perception has an important impact on the effectiveness of communication processes.

5.1 Defining communication

In communication science and related disciplines, several conceptual models have been developed to reflect the communication process. For many years, communication was defined in terms of 'information transfer', i.e. 'the process of sending and receiving messages through channels, which establishes common meanings between source and receiver' (*cf.* van den Ban & Hawkins, 1996). Sender and receiver can change roles, whereby the original sender receives feedback from the original receiver through a similar communication procedure. This definition is illustrated in Berlo's (1960) so-called 'Source, Message, Channel, Receiver, Effect-model' (Figure 5.1). This SMCRE-model suggests that the received information is the same as the information that has been transferred by the sender. However, it often appears that a receiver arrives at an interpretation that differs from the meaning as intended by the sender. In such situations the result of the communication process is ineffective: sender and receiver do not manage to establish a common meaning. Researchers and practitioners came to realise the limitations of this linear representation of the communication process. In section 3.1 we explained why people can

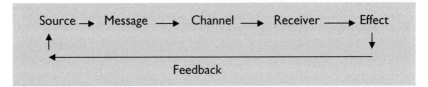

Figure 5.1 The SMCRE-model.

differ in their interpretations. People's perceptions are relative, selective, and organised and stored in mental sets. It is not too difficult to understand that these mental sets influence the communication process. Two additional elements are essential in understanding causes of distortion in the communication process: symbols and meaning, and the processes of encoding and decoding.

5.1.1 Symbols and meaning

Communicated messages consist of symbols and meaning. *Symbols* are physical elements that are important for both source and receiver. They may be verbal or nonverbal, auditory, such as tone of voice, or visual, such as signs, gestures or drawings. It can be speech or writing, a smile or a gesture, a laugh or a hand on a shoulder. A symbol has no meaning by itself. It is given *meaning* by the people who use it or see it. As Berlo (1960) says, 'Meanings are in people'. This generalisation has important consequences for communication. People sometimes attach a different meaning to the same stimuli. Take the word 'volunteer'. To most people a volunteer is someone who undertakes a task spontaneously, but for a botanist or agronomist a volunteer is a seed that germinates spontaneously. Messages are interpreted within the frame of reference of the receiver. This frame is based on pre-existing knowledge and on personal history: the culture in which one has grown up, and the norms and values that have been learned both within the family and at school. In addition, factors such as politics, social relationships, emotions, interests, and aspirations are part of this frame of reference. If we are not aware of these frames of reference, we easily fall into the trap known as *the fallacy of the empty vessel*. The chances of health communicators being effective are low if they think that all they have to do to ensure the success of their programme is to pour health information into the minds of the population. The frame of reference of this population influences successful communication.

5.1.2 Encoding and decoding

Encoding is the cognitive process of transforming ideas and feelings into symbols, and subsequently organising them into a message. *Decoding* is the process of transforming the message of another back into one's own ideas and feelings (Verderber, 1996). These processes are actually the basics for communication. Encoding and decoding are not limited to language. The processes are to a large extent influenced by nonverbal cues. In situations in which the receiver observes the sender (this may be a real life observation or based on filmed images), the most important nonverbal cues are derived from body language. This includes facial expressions, gestures, tone of voice, and pose. For instance, if your colleague says: 'I really appreciate your opinion on this matter', the meaning you decode will be very different if the person looks interestedly in your direction or if the person looks away. Nonverbal communication may be *complementary* to verbal communication. For instance, the sender can accentuate the importance of a message by means of gestures, raised tone of voice, or a pause before saying something important. Nonverbal cues can also *contradict* verbal communication. A hostile voice contradicts friendly words. Nonverbal communication can also *substitute* verbal communication. From a person's appearance alone we can derive whether this person is happy or sad, and from a facial expression we can derive if a person agrees or disagrees with what we say. Encoding and decoding are also influenced by relationships. According to Watzlawick *et al.* (1967), communication contains a 'content' and a 'relational' aspect. Content refers to what is said literally, the relational aspect to what it *does* to the relationship between the communicating partners. For example, a father asking his son 'Can you please close the door?' may really want his son to close the door, but may in fact also be commanding his son to leave the room.

In everyday life, communication, encoding and decoding are subconscious processes. Only in specific situations, for example if we want to make a certain idea very clear, do we think consciously about choice of words, gestures that support the idea, etcetera. But even when a person consciously encodes a message to create a specific meaning, the decoding person may receive a meaning that differs from what the encoder thought he or she was communicating. Consider the example of the 'volunteer'. Thus, in communication we do not simply transfer ideas from person to person. *We elicit meanings.* The source of an idea encodes his or her thoughts in a message, which may consist of both verbal and nonverbal cues, and which is subsequently decoded or interpreted by the receiver. This process can result in a shared meaning. However, because source and receiver do not always share common meanings for words, symbols and gestures, the process can also result in different meanings.

5.1.3 Redefining communication

Insights into the processes of encoding and decoding, and the factors influencing these processes, have led to a refined definition of communication. Communication is no longer defined in terms of a linear process, but as *the transactional process of creating meaning* (*cf.* Watzlawick *et al.*, 1967; Wilmot, 1987; DeVito, 1994). The main difference between this definition and the one given previously lies in the word 'transactional'. Transactional means that communication is interactive, and that those communicating are mutually responsible for the meaning that each creates during and after the interaction. In composing and interpreting a message, both source and receiver use their own frame of reference. This process is presented in Figure 5.2.

The probability of unintended meanings is reduced if the sender is receiver-oriented, that is, if the sender makes an effort to understand the frame of reference of the receiver. Moreover, the sender can use the feedback from the receiver to decide whether or not the message has been interpreted correctly. This latter, however, is more difficult if there is no feedback or direct contact between sender and receiver, e.g. in communication through a mass medium as this book.

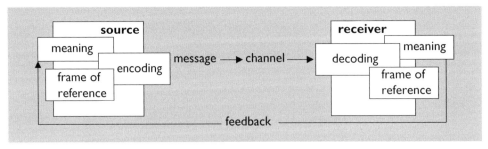

Figure 5.2 The communication process.

5.2 Purposes of communication

Communication always has - consciously or subconsciously - a purpose. DeVito (1994) describes five major purposes of communication. We mention them only briefly here. For a more detailed description, refer to DeVito (1994:17-20). General purposes of communication are (a) to discover: learn about oneself and the other person; (b) to relate: to establish and maintain close relationships with others; (c) to help: therapists, counsellors, parents and friends are just a few categories of those who often communicate to help; (d) to persuade: both interpersonally and through mass media we seek to change attitudes and behaviours; and (e) to play: to tell jokes, say clever things, and relate interesting stories largely for the pleasure it gives oneself and the listener. Of course this list is not complete and, in addition, communication acts are usually motivated by a combination of purposes.

5.2.1 Purposes of health communication

The five general purposes of communication are actually purposes for health communication as well. However, when we design health communication interventions, three major purposes can be identified: to inform, to persuade and to educate (*cf.* van Woerkum *et al.*, 1999). *Informational communication* refers to the conscious communication of information to help people to form sound opinions and make good decisions (van den Ban & Hawkins, 1996). Informational communication is aimed at people who only have a need for specific information to make decisions, are well capable of elaborating on that information, and are capable of making choices (van Woerkum *et al.*, 1999). For example, if you plan to go on holiday, you are perhaps looking for information about your destination in order to decide about short trips. Or consider the example of someone who has decided to change dietary habits and is looking for low-fat recipes. The aim of informational communication thus is 'to inform'. The communication is effective if it indeed facilitates the receiver in forming opinions and making decisions. *Persuasive communication* differs in this respect. With persuasive communication we purposefully try to persuade - to convince - the receiver to change attitudes, goals and behaviour in a predefined direction. Commercial advertising and political propaganda, for example, use such persuasive strategies, but a lot of health communication is also based on persuasion. Just consider the efforts to convince people to wear seatbelts, to change dietary habits, or to practice safe sex. Persuasive communication can be a delicate activity though, since the implicit or explicit message is that there is something wrong with the way the receiver is currently thinking or acting. There is, however, a major difference between health communication and others forms of persuasive communication: who benefits? The benefits of successful marketing and propaganda accrue finally to the sender, whereas the benefits of effective persuasive health communication usually accrue to the receivers. In addition, the benefits can accrue to a collective good, for example, to prevent the spreading of contagious diseases or to decrease the costs of poor health. We therefore wish to define *persuasive health communication* as a professional communication intervention to induce change in a voluntary behaviour with a presumed individual, public or collective utility (*cf.* Koelen & Martijn, 1994; Röling, 1988; also see section 2.2). *Educational communication* again is different. The focus is not on 'wrong attitudes' or 'wrong practices', but on helping people to identify their own needs, to improve their problem solving capacity, and to gain skills and self confidence to act upon their needs. Educational communication is based on the notion that 'it is better to teach someone how to catch fish, than to provide him with a fish everyday' (*cf.* Heymann, 1994). In fact, Tschajanov, a Russian agronomist, already advocated this approach in 1917. In his opinion, in agricultural extension the focus should not be on telling farmers what to do, but on enhancing their capacity to make their own decisions (Tschajanow, 1924). Educational communication is closely related to what we called the participatory approach in section 2.2, and its purpose is closely related to the objectives of health promotion, i.e. empowerment.

The three purposes of health communication are not mutually exclusive. On the contrary. In practice they are often intermingled: in persuasive communication we also provide information to facilitate decision making, and educational communication often contains persuasive elements as well. Quite often too, the different strategies are used in chronological order. For example, at the outset of the HIV/AIDS epidemic communications were almost purely persuasive, trying to create awareness and to convince populations of the importance of preventive behaviours. The second flow of communication was more informative, so as to provide information about possibilities for prevention. Subsequently, communicative interventions focused on how to bring preventive sexual behaviour into practice. Hence, it was more educational in nature.

5.3 Source, message, channel, and receiver

As we pointed out in section 5.1, source, message, channel and receiver influence the outcomes of communicative interventions. In communication science and related disciplines, an enormous amount of research is focused on these elements. In this section we present some of the insights from that research.

5.3.1 Source

Characteristics of the source of a message play an important role in the effectiveness of communication. Credibility, attractiveness, likeability, and the power of the communicator have been shown to affect the outcome of communication processes. *Credibility* refers to judgements made by a receiver concerning the believability of a communicator. Communicator credibility is not intrinsic. While it may be a characteristic of the communicator (e.g. a medical doctor will be seen as a credible source for health information), it is not the only criterion a receiver uses to judge credibility. If the same medical doctor talks about football, he may not be seen as a credible source. A message source may be seen as highly credible by one receiver and not at all by another. For example, a young mother may be a credible source for another young mother, but not for a teenage girl. Credibility is largely determined by the perceived competence and perceived trustworthiness of the communicator. If both are high, the receiver is more prone to accept the message than if one or both of them is low. *Likeability* refers to the extent to which the receiver likes the communicator. Research shows that, in general, liked communicators are more effective than disliked communicators. Likeability of the source is especially important if the receiver's involvement in the subject is low (I like this person, so I will agree). The effects of likeability decrease if the involvement of the receiver increases. Finally, the *power* of the source can influence the acceptance of a message. When a source can distribute or control rewards and punishments, such as grants, rebates or recognition, the receiver will be more prone to behave in the advised direction.

5.3.2 Message

The message refers to what is said and how it is said. Important aspects of messages are content, strategy, and language. *Message content* refers to the advocated position and the arguments that substantiate that position. The discrepancy between the position advocated in the message and the receiver's position influences the effectiveness of a message. In general it is found that minor discrepancies are more effective in inducing behaviour change than larger discrepancies. Extremely discrepant messages are readily ignored by the receiver (Sherif & Hovland, 1961; Sherif, 1980; also see section 5.4.1). Other studies have shown that messages that stimulate thinking, messages that contain strong arguments, or messages that add something new to what is already known, are more likely to be accepted (Petty & Cacioppo, 1984; Leippe & Elkin, 1987). Moreover, people may offer more resistance to messages that make a direct appeal to change behaviour than to messages with a hidden agenda. Thus, we are less likely to reject cleverly devised television commercials in which actors portray behaviour desired by the advertiser than we are to reject more direct appeals for us to change our behaviour. The level of complexity of a message is also crucial. In general, it is preferable to use simple, easy-to-comprehend messages. This may be difficult, because health-related issues are sometimes quite complicated.

Message strategy includes the tenor or purport of the message, fear appeals, and the use of emotional versus factual information. By *tenor* we mean whether the message addresses the unhealthy behaviour or its healthy counterparts, and whether it is positively or negatively phrased. For example, in stimulating people to give up smoking we can focus either on the advantages of not smoking, or on the disadvantages of continuing to smoke. There is ample evidence that, in the long run, positive expressions are more appealing than negative expressions.

In the area of persuasive communication, a lot of research has been devoted to the effects of fear appeals. As we have seen in section 3.6, fear can be an important motive for behaviour change. Health communication often conveys such fear appeals - for example, television clips showing gruesome traffic accidents caused by drunk drivers in an effort to discourage such dangerous practices, or stop-smoking messages displaying lungs affected by cancer. Research shows that increases in fear are associated with increases in acceptance of the message, increasing the chances of change in intentions and behaviour (for a comprehensive overview, see Sutton, 1982). Several researchers also suggest that the persuasive effectiveness decreases if the levels of fear arousal are too high, but results are not unambiguous to this point (Reardon, 1991).

An additional point to consider in relation to message strategy is whether to make the message rational, presenting relatively straightforward factual information, or to dramatise the message. The dramatic approach is likely to have more emotional appeal and may reach a wider audience than the factual approach. Research evidence shows that, when the information in the arguments is important and unfamiliar to the audience, the emphasis should be on rational arguments. When importance is low and familiarity is high, emotional appeals are more effective. Emotional appeals, which stimulate discussion among their audience, have a high probability of changing behaviour. H. Beecher Stowe's book *Uncle Tom's Cabin* (1852) probably had more influence on the abolition of slavery in the United States than any unemotional and purely factual presentation might have had.

In addition to the abovementioned variables, *language* needs consideration. Health communicators with specific technical expertise are often bound to a certain terminology that is familiar to them and hence assume this terminology is familiar to everyone. For example, in nutrition education we often see such words as cholesterol, staple foods, proteins, etc. People, however, do not use these nutrient categories when they think about food. It is not in their frame of reference. They consume such products as potatoes, butter, eggs, carrots or apples. We also have to be aware of differences in language used by different social groups. For example, teenagers use different words and phrases than adults to express what is of value to them, and so on.

So far, our discussion has assumed that one sender communicates with one receiver. However, usually the reality is more complicated. Both sender and receiver are often at the same time influenced by their social environment, the family to which they belong, their friends, their colleagues, etc. One implication of this is that the receiver receives messages not only from the sender, but at the same time from other people in the social environment. The receiver will be aware that those people have certain opinions and expectations with regard to which ideas are correct and which behaviour is proper. Consider what we said about social influence in section 3.7. For a sender it may be very difficult to realise changes in knowledge and/or attitudes that makes the receiver a deviant in his or her social environment. It is, for instance, difficult to convince a girl that she should refrain from taking up smoking, when she aspires to belong to a group in which nearly everyone smokes. The result may be that she is expelled from this group, which can be considered as a serious social punishment. We return to this communication problem in section 6.2.5.

5.3.3 Channel

The word 'channel' refers to the way in which the message is transferred. In health communication we can use a variety of ways to bring about the message. The methods can be placed in a dimension ranging from a merely one-way flow of information, as is the case with the conventional mass media - such as television, radio or print - to an active two-way exchange, as is the case in a face-to-face interaction between two individuals, i.e. interpersonal communication. Interpersonal communication can be further divided in mediated and non-mediated communication. *Mediated communication* refers to all types of communication processes where face-to-face communication is mediated by technical devices, for example telephone, electronic mail messages, video conferencing or letters (Wallbott, 1996). Non-mediated communication refers to any type of face-to-face communication in which the parties interact at the same time and in the same place, without a technical device. Between the extremes we can place methods that contain some aspects of both, such as lectures (one speaker to an audience), demonstrations, and group discussions. An additional type of media that typically possesses some of the characteristics of mass media and some characteristics of interpersonal communication is referred to as 'hybrid media', that is, media based in computer and information technology (ICT) (see Figure 5.3).

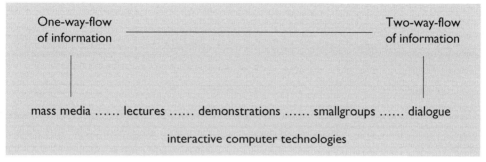

Figure 5.3 Dimension of information flows.

The processes of influence through different communication channels differ from each other in three important ways. The first difference is the extent to which receivers are free to interpret or decode a message according to their own views. For example, a receiver who decodes a non-illustrated article about a country he or she has never visited will probably end up with a different image of the country than a receiver who sees a television report showing the life of people in that country. Secondly, there is a difference in the extent to which feedback is possible. Face-to-face communication offers far greater opportunities for feedback than a radio broadcast. The third variable is the extent to which receivers are influenced by their own group membership. Group influence is much stronger when receivers are participating in a discussion than when they are reading about the same issue in a magazine or leaflet.

It should be realised that, while message content may be held constant across channels, different communication modes often vary in the way the message is perceived and interpreted. Research of Chaiken and Eagly (1976), for example, has shown that easy messages in easy-to-understand language are clearly understood, whether they are presented in a printed version, on an audiotape or videotape. Difficult messages in technical language, however, limit the comprehension of the receivers if presented as speech, but not if they were presented in printed form. According to Zimbardo and Leippe (1991), this makes sense, since while reading one can re-read and pause to contemplate and assimilate information, and so cut through technical jargon. Several other points have to be considered when choosing a channel, for example the size of the audience, the extent to which an individual is involved in the activities associated with the message, the nature of the audience, and the costs per person reached. In Chapter 6 we discuss in more detail the ways in which messages can be transferred.

5.3.4 Receiver

The receiver of a message has some characteristics that are important for the results of the communication process. Receivers' communication skills, attitudes, knowledge, self-efficacy, and social background influence how they receive and interpret a message. Previously we referred to this as a person's frame of reference. Involvement or the personal relevance of the topic also plays an important role. Changes in opinions, attitudes or behaviour through communication are often based on careful consideration (elaboration) of the pros and cons associated with the advocated position, but they can also occur based on peripheral cues. These latter cues seem to be important when there is little interest in the subject, or a lack of ability or motivation to evaluate the message (Petty & Cacioppo, 1986; Chaiken, 1987). Demographic characteristics and capacity variables such as gender, ethnicity, age, and education also have an influence.

5.4 Other factors influencing effective communication

In the foregoing sections we presented a model of the communication process, and we discussed the influence of source, message, channel, and receiver on the outcomes of communicative interventions. The model gives a basic understanding of communication processes and is helpful in developing health communication programmes and strategies. There are, however, a few types of problems that may exist in sending and receiving messages and which influence the effectiveness of the communication. In 5.4.1 we discuss the influence of selectivity, and in 5.4.2 some additional problems.

5.4.1 Selectivity

In section 3.1 we briefly discussed the concept of selectivity, i.e. the tendency of individuals to pay attention to only a selection of the stimuli surrounding us. Selective perception can be defined as the conscious or unconscious increase in attention to stimuli and information consistent with a person's attitudes or interests, or conscious or unconscious discounting of inconsistent stimuli (Dictionary of Marketing Terms, 2004). In general, we use selective perception to protect ourselves from the chaos and confusion of excessive and conflicting incoming stimuli. Two types of selective perception are of special importance for health communication: selective attention and selective acceptance.

Selective attention
Nobody can read everything that is published or hear everything that is communicated, so we must select rigorously. In relation to the notion of a 'person's interest' in the abovementioned definition, people generally only pay attention to information that is somehow relevant to them. Likewise, people are prone to ignore or neglect information about subjects in which they are not interested. For instance, there is a lot of information available about computers, but we may not be aware of all this information until we intend to buy one. In health education we often provide information about subjects in which people are not directly interested. It seems reasonable to argue that mere exposure does not elicit attention to the message. Gaining attention is crucial, but also difficult. Batra and Ray (1983) summarise findings from research on learning as a result of advertising exposure. They conclude that only a small proportion of advertising messages receive attention. 'With a typical family being exposed to well over 1,000 messages a day, only those that are stronger (louder, brighter, larger, etc.) than others, different (but not too different so as not to be rejected as strange) and of interest or value - have potential for receiving attention' (Batra & Ray, 1983:129). As we argued in section 4.1, the first step in the innovation decision process is awareness, which requires that people are exposed to the information (McGuire, 1985), and that they pay attention to it. It means that the message, next to being conspicuous, must elicit feelings that the information being presented in the message has something interesting to say.

In relation to the notion of a 'person's attitude', selective attention refers to the tendency to pay closer attention to a message that supports one's existing attitude or opinion than to a message that opposes it. Several studies have been conducted in which subjects are exposed to a message containing an equal number of arguments pro and contra the receiver's opinion. Generally, the results show that the subjects do pick out the supporting arguments in preference to the opposing ones. In a classical review of literature on selective exposure, Sears and Freedman (1971) concluded that people indeed tend to expose themselves to information with which they agree. Possible reasons for selection are the usefulness of the information, the need to solve certain problems, the need to participate in discussions with friends or to confirm one's own point of view, as well as to avoid dissonance. According to Festinger (1957), cognitive dissonance results from receiving information that opposes one's beliefs, attitudes, or opinions. Dissonance is a psychologically uncomfortable situation, as unpleasant as, for example, anxiety. Thus, people are motivated to reduce dissonance and achieve consonance. When dissonance is present, in addition to trying to reduce it, the person will actively avoid situations and information that are likely to increase dissonance (Festinger, 1957). It is perhaps for this reason that smokers, for example, cover up the warnings on cigarette packages, and that people practising unprotected sex believe that they are invulnerable to sexually transmittable diseases, contrary to the available evidence.

Selective acceptance
Even if people pay attention to messages, they do not generally accept everything they hear or read. For instance, we may remember advertisements telling us that Brand A washing powder is more effective than any other brand, but we do not *believe* the content of this advertisement. We tend to accept ideas more easily when they agree with our own opinions. Interesting in this respect is the notion that has been spelled out in the social judgement theory (Sherif *et al.*, 1965; Sherif, 1980). According to this theory, the effect of communication depends on how a receiver evaluates the position advocated in a message. A receiver will evaluate the position advocated in a message using his or her own position as a point of reference: 'the most acceptable position'. The position advocated in a message, and the receiver's initial position, can be placed on a so-called judgement scale (see Figure 5.4). The theory uses the term 'range of positions' to indicate that people generally find more positions acceptable than the one exactly matching their own stand on the issue. They also find more positions objectionable. A person will accept a range of positions located around his or her most preferred position. This is called the *latitude of acceptance*. The range of positions that the receiver finds unacceptable is called the *latitude of rejection*. Between the acceptable and

unacceptable positions, there is a range of positions the receiver neither accepts nor rejects: the *latitude of non-commitment*. The range can be large (e.g. five positions on the scale), or small (e.g. two positions). According to the theory, the size of the range is influenced by the receiver's level of involvement with the issue. Higher levels of involvement coincide with decreased latitudes of acceptance and non-commitment, and increased latitudes of rejection. Low levels of involvement coincide with increased latitudes of acceptance and non-commitment, and a decrease in the latitude of rejection. The structure of the judgmental latitudes will vary from person to person. Hence, two people with the same 'most acceptable position' may differ in their latitudes of acceptance, rejection and non-commitment. Consider for example a message advocating a moderate pro-abortion position. The message is sent to two receivers, each with a moderate con-position as an anchor point. For one reason or another, receiver A is more involved in the issue than receiver B. How will they react to the message? Figure 5.4 shows the position of both receivers on the judgement scale, and we see that the range of the three areas differs for both receivers. For receiver A, the latitude of acceptance and the latitude of non-commitment are smaller than for receiver B, and the latitude of rejection is larger. We also see that the position advocated in the messages falls into receiver B's latitude of acceptance, but into A's latitude of rejection. Generally, if a message falls into the latitude of

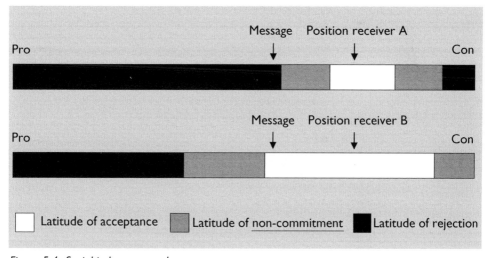

Figure 5.4 Social judgement scale.

rejection, the receiver will reject or even ignore the message. Most change can be expected if the message takes a position with a small discrepancy in relation to the most preferred position, but which still lies within the latitude of acceptance. Hence, receiver A will reject the message and will not think about it. Receiver B, on the other hand, will accept the message and think about the contents.

In this judgmental process, two distortions may appear: assimilation or contrast. *Assimilation* refers to the false perception that a message advocates the same position as the receiver holds, as a consequence of which the receiver does not pay any attention to the actual content ('nothing new'). *Contrast*, on the other hand, refers to the false perception that the position advocated in the message is so different from his or her own position that the receiver ignores it ('this is not meant for me'). It is clear that both effects lead to ineffective communication. Assimilation and contrast effects are minimised if the advocated position in the message is made very clear.

5.4.2 Additional problems in effective health communication

In addition to selectivity, we have to consider some natural, sociological and psychological factors that affect the effectiveness of health communication. Here we will briefly elaborate on unhealthy attractions, unrealistic optimism, probabilistic outcomes, cynicism about health messages, and dealing with opposing messages. *Unhealthy attractions* refer to the strength of existing attitudes and habits that the message seeks to change. People often enjoy existing habits, such as smoking, sweets, and even altered states of consciousness. Mere messages may be insufficient to change strong, and possibly desirable, habits (Zimbardo & Leippe, 1991). *Unrealistic optimism* refers to the fact that the average person sees him or herself as 'above average' in general health, and 'below average' in the risk of disease, injury, and premature death. This phenomenon is also referred to as optimism bias (see Weinstein 1987; 1989). Van de Velde *et al.* (1994), for example, asked a random sample of persons to estimate both their own chances of becoming infected with the AIDS virus within the next two years because of their sexual behaviour and the chances of a man/woman of their own age doing so. They found that subjects estimated their own risk as being much lower (five per cent) than the risk for others (19 per cent). As Zimbardo and Leippe (1991:343) argue, optimism about one's health and an illusion of personal invulnerability are nice defences against anxiety and worry; but if *over*-optimism is the rule, many of us may fail to perceive the self-relevance of important health advice, and hence fail to systematically analyse it. *Probabilistic outcomes* refer to the uncertainty of the outcomes of behaviour change. Engaging in health protective behaviour reduces, but does not eliminate, the risk of disease. A healthy diet, for example, is no safeguard against cardiovascular diseases. Moreover, only a few health-related behaviours have an immediate and noticeable effect on health. On the contrary, the outcome is often long term. For the less healthy behaviours, this relation is reversed: rewards are short term (e.g. the pleasure of smoking a cigarette is immediate), and possible negative consequences (e.g. lung cancer) are long term. Generally, short-term rewards are more powerful influences than the probability of long-term health gains. *Cynicism about health messages* is another obstacle to effective health communication. Endless bad news about disease-causing habits (e.g. coffee, tea, sweets, salt, high levels of cholesterol, fatty foods that contribute to heart disease or cancers) may compel people to tune out health messages. Finally, health messages must often *compete with opposing messages*. Industry promotes its products in an attractive manner. Think of advertisements for alcoholic beverages, cigarettes, candies, and many other pleasurable and tasty goods. As we mentioned before, positive messages are generally more accepted than negative ones. Health messages often point to negative consequences of such pleasures. In addition, opposing information stems not only from media messages, but also from influential sources surrounding us, such as peers, family members or colleagues. Even between health organisations, messages are not always consistent. For example, one professional organisation may advise the eating of no more than two eggs per week, whereas the other organisation advocates the position that three eggs is the maximum. There is a general tendency in individuals to ignore opposing or contradictory messages, as a result of which people stick to their existing conduct.

5.5 Chapter summary

In this chapter we defined communication as the transactional process of creating meaning. The result of this process depends on the way in which verbal and nonverbal symbols are encoded by the sender, and decoded by the receiver. We discussed several aspects that may reduce or increase the effectiveness of communication. These relate to characteristics of the source, the message, the channel, and the receiver. Moreover, selective perception and selective acceptance are important aspects influencing the effectiveness of communication. All these aspects have to be considered when designing health messages. This is based on one of the premises of effective communication, that is, that one has to know the audience and the audience's frame of reference. Insight into existing opinions and preferences is necessary, since these guide the processes of selectivity. We often try to expose target groups to information they have not asked for, in which they are not interested, and which is inconsistent with their existing opinions and behaviour. If we do not take these aspects into account, the receivers will be inclined either not to notice the message, or to openly ignore or reject it.

6. Media and methods for health communication

In this chapter we point out some of the approaches commonly used in health communication. The choice of any one of the methods available will depend on the specific goals and on the circumstances in which they are applied. In Chapter 5, we positioned communication methods on a dimension ranging from one-way information to one-to-one communications (see Figure 5.3). Conventional mass media, positioned on the left extreme, are characterised by an absence of direct interaction with the audience. The further the methods move to the right, the more interpersonal communication becomes, with face-to-face, non-mediated, interaction on the right extreme. In this chapter, we elaborate on the different media and discuss their strengths and weaknesses. Firstly, we address the conventional mass media (e.g. television, radio, and newspapers) and also pay some attention to specifically designed print mass media, i.e. posters and leaflets. We then proceed with interpersonal methods (dialogue, lectures, demonstrations, and small group methods). Finally we elaborate to some extent on hybrid media (World Wide Web, online support groups, and computer tailoring). We end this chapter with a brief discussion about how different methods can be combined into one programme.

6.1 Conventional mass media

Mass media include all media where the communication process is public, diverse, indirect, via a technical medium, basically one-sided, and usually addressed to a large and more or less anonymous audience (Harris, 1989). Examples are radio, television, and print media. The primary purpose of those mass media is not to serve a public health goal, but to bring news or entertainment. Whereas 'man bites dog' would attract attention as news, 'dog bites man' would be regarded as too commonplace to warrant media attention. Nevertheless, health-related issues receive considerable attention in the news media. For example, *Media Monitor* (1997) reports that in the course of the 1990s news about health and medicine was the third largest topic in the USA evening news shows, just after topics on crime and economic news. In the year 2000, health news held the forth position, due to the fact that the number one position was held by news on the presidential elections at that time (*Media Monitor*, 2001). For local television news, health is the fifth most common news (CMPA Archive, 1996). Coverage tends to focus on new discoveries about diseases or their treatment. In discussions about diseases, cancer received most attention, followed by heart disease, AIDS and Alzheimer's disease (*Media Monitor*, 2001). However, disease prevention, health behaviour (e.g. diet, physical activity and smoking), or early detection for disease prevention receives hardly any attention (Caburnay *et al.*, 2003). These are examples of media coverage directed by the 'newsmakers'. The public mass media are, however, increasingly used for the transmission of specific health education campaigns as well. In many countries, governmental and non-governmental organisations buy media time to broadcast short television ads around popular programmes at prime time, for instance anti-smoking campaigns, campaigns to promote seatbelt use, to promote safe sex, to lower fat intake, or to refrain from drinking alcohol when driving.

An interesting possibility for using public mass media is found in what is called entertainment-education. *Entertainment-education* can be defined as: 'the process of purposely designing and implementing a media message both to entertain and educate, in order to increase audience members' knowledge about an educational issue, create favourable attitudes, and change overt behaviour' (*cf.* Singhal & Rogers, 1999:9). The approach draws upon Bandura's (1986) social learning theory. According to this theory, people can learn by observing and imitating the behaviour of others in real life or on film or television (vicarious learning; also see section 3.2). The idea of integrating educational messages and amusement is not new. Storytelling, theatre, poems and songs have been used for both entertainment and educational purposes for thousands of years. In the past three decades, its power seems to have been rediscovered. An increasing number of soap operas, game shows and cartoons contain a combination of entertainment and education (*cf.* Bouman, 1999). The most widely known example is Sesame Street, a television series that helps prepare preschool children for classroom learning. The series is broadcast in more than 140 countries on six continents (*Children's Television Workshop*, 1998). Entertainment has the potential to reach larger audiences than news (Finnigan & Viswanath,

1999). Moreover, it can provide health messages in an attractive and interesting format. Entertainment-education has been successfully applied to a variety of issues, such as racial and ethnic prejudice, child abuse, drunk driving, drug abuse, nutrition and cardiovascular disease, sexually transmittable diseases such as HIV/AIDS, and family planning (for an extensive overview, refer to Singhal & Rogers, 1999; 2003). Based on the existing evidence, we can say that using entertainment to carry health messages appears to be a promising strategy for the use of mass media in public health campaigns.

Posters and leaflets
Posters and leaflets are examples of printed mass media which are specifically designed to communicate specific health-related issues, for example, a leaflet presenting '10 rules for a healthy diet', a leaflet containing practical information about breast self-examination, or a poster promoting condom use. We specifically address these forms of mass media because their use is popular and widespread. Leaflets and posters are often used as 'stand alone' mass media, but they can also be used in addition to interpersonal forms of communication. *Posters* mainly have an attention drawing function. They are limited as to the amount of information they can contain. Usually people will not stop to read complicated texts on a poster. This means that the message has to be clear at first glance, it has to be appealing, and it has to stimulate the viewer to think about the content of the message. Posters can function as an *introduction to interpersonal communication*. For example, in a campaign aimed at reducing the incidence of baby bottle caries, parents of young children were advised to change from using a feeding bottle to using a cup when the child was about nine months old. Posters containing the short message: 'Bottle it up, take a cup' were placed in the waiting rooms of well-baby clinics. The paediatrician in an interpersonal consultation addressed the issue. Interviews with parents showed that, if they had seen the poster, they were more prepared to discuss the issue with the paediatrician than those who had not seen it (*cf.* Koelen *et al.*, 2000). *Leaflets* can have a meaningful function *following interpersonal communication*. Leaflets can contain more information than posters and enable the receiver to re-read the information at his or her own pace, and at the moment she or he has a need for this information. It should be considered however that, even though the use of leaflets is widespread, research also shows that receivers often report not receiving them, not remembering them or,

if they do remember them, not reading them. Clearly, the use of leaflets on their own is less effective, but used in combination with interpersonal communication leaflets seem to enhance the effects of such communication.

6.1.1 Effects of conventional mass media

Different opinions have been expressed about the extent to which the mass media influence people's thoughts and actions. Mass media, especially newspaper, radio and television, have the image of being powerful. For example, authoritarian governments, both in the past and at present, often try to control those mass media, based on the notion that they can selectively influence the ways people think and see reality, to prevent others from presenting a different point of view. The actual strength of the mass media in influencing people has for a long time already been a topic of discussion. In the 1950s, several reports were published which showed that the media had limited influence. Later it was assumed that the mass media are more influential than it was thought in the 1950s (*cf.* Windahl *et al.,* 1991). The many discussions about the influence of the mass media, and specifically the influence of television and movies, on aggression and prejudice indeed indicate that some consider the influence of the mass media to be strong and direct. Likewise, the expected strong influence of mass media cigarette advertisements, and the current ban on such ads in many European countries and the USA, indicate that the mass media are considered powerful. At the same time, several authors have argued that the influence of the mass media is mainly indirect (*cf.* Klapper, 1960; McGuire, 1985; van Woerkum, 1999), that is, the mass media serve primarily to put things on the agenda for further discussion among an audience. The question of how much influence the mass media actually have is to date far from resolved. As Wallbott (1996:319) expresses it, the discussion seems to oscillate between the view that the media have no direct impact at all, and if there is an influence it is mediated via personal communication with opinion leaders, and the opposite view that the mass media are our central source of knowledge, that they determine our view of the world, and, consequently, our behaviour. No doubt, however, the mass media fulfil certain functions in our societies and in changing these societies. These functions include setting the agenda of important discussion topics; transferring knowledge; forming and changing opinions; and changing behaviour.

Agenda setting refers to the ability of the media to select and call to the public's attention both ideas and events (Agee *et al.*, 1988). They put things on the agenda, and they have an influence on *what* people talk about. Indeed, research shows a strong relation between what the public believes to be important issues and issues that are actually covered by the media (*cf.* Behr & Iyengar, 1985; Kasperson, 1988; Frewer *et al.*, 2002). Good examples are the huge mass media attention on HIV/AIDS in the late 1980s, or the attention on genetic modification of food and mad cow disease (BSE) in Europe in the late 1990s, issues which at that time were real topics for public debate. There are, however, two points to consider. Firstly, media have an influence on *what* people talk about, but not on *how* they talk about it. This largely depends on the context in which messages are received, including the receiver's values and norms, and those of the social environment of which he or she is part (i.e. frame of reference). Moreover, people are not passive recipients of information (see section 3.1 and 3.2). They actively think about what they hear and see, they talk about it with others, they shape, alter and recreate the message, and they process and interpret the message in the context of their frame of reference. Consequently, different receivers will come to different conclusions and interpretations. For example, media attention on HIV/AIDS has led to massive public discussion about preventing further spread of the disease. But different parties involved in these discussions have come to different conclusions: some advocating the promotion of safe sex, others advocating monogamy and virginity until marriage. Secondly, media attention can lead to hypes, that is, an issue suddenly gets media attention which leads to intensified public concern, which in turn leads to intensified media attention, etc., and then the media attention disappears as suddenly as it came (van Ginneken, 1999). Kasperson (1988) refers to this phenomenon as 'social amplification'. Consider again the example of HIV/AIDS. In the early 1980s, the disease attracted massive media attention. Each 'new case' was extensively reported. Currently however, media attention on HIV/AIDS is almost non-existent, even though in many countries, especially developing countries, it is a major cause of death.

Despite such considerations, the mass media have to be considered as a strong and useful instrument. How well the mass media function on behalf of public health goals is significantly influenced by how well the field of public health itself manages to engage the media (Finnegan &

Viswanath, 1999; Bouman, 1999). Radio and TV programme designers and print media editors will certainly be interested in covering health issues if they consider the subject interesting and important for their audience. According to Aarts (1998), the timing and framing of mass media messages are important issues to consider when the purpose is to set public agendas. By putting things on the agenda, the media can raise public awareness and promote greater consideration or public discourse about individual, social or policy issues. In addition, mass media can have an important function in the *diffusion* and acquisition of new information and knowledge. It should be noted, however, that such knowledge is more likely to be transferred successfully if it meets a need or fills a vacuum. New ideas diffused through the media are more acceptable if they link up with existing knowledge (see section 5.4). Related to agenda setting and knowledge transfer, the mass media may play an important role in *developing opinions*, especially when the audience does not have strong views about a particular issue. The media can have important effects in *changing opinions* as well, especially when the position advocated in the message differs only slightly from the receiver's own opinions (see section 5.4). If an issue is considered important, people are inclined to think about it more carefully, and to find out what other people think, before they make up their own minds. Others may take the initiative in these discussions if they think the subject to be important enough. It should be noted that opinions expressed in the media are not always unanimous, and sometimes even contradictory. As we argued before, people in this situation are inclined to ignore the contradictory information, and to decide not to change opinions. Mass media campaigns usually have weak effects on actual health *behaviours*. Just consider the numbers of mass media anti-smoking campaigns. Nevertheless, under specific conditions, mass media campaigns can have a function in *changing behaviour*, particularly where these changes are small and easy to conduct. An item on the eight o'clock news saying that shrimps are contaminated with the salmonella bacteria, and recommending that people do not consume shrimps for the next three weeks, will have an enormous effect. For more complicated issues, such as giving up smoking or losing weight, the mass media can provide arguments, but these will not be strong enough to induce an actual change of these habits.

Taking into account the possible effects, we can conclude that the conventional mass media are important in the first stage of the innovation decision process (see section 4.1), but that their influence decreases in the later stages. Tones and Tilford (1994) refer in this regard to a 'hierarchy of effects'. It is relatively easy to set an agenda and to communicate simple information, but it is increasingly difficult to change attitudes, teach complex skills and persuade people to adopt new behaviours. The mass media can support, and in some cases accelerate, existing change processes, but they seldom bring about changes in behaviour by themselves.

6.1.2 Mass media choice by receivers

The ways in which people use different mass media have been studied frequently in industrialised countries. In general, there is an increasing tendency to spend more time with television and radio than with the printed word. Media exposure does not occur equally across all social groups. People with higher formal education (as a measure of socio-economic status: SES) pay more attention to print media, especially magazines, and less to television than people with lower educational levels. People with higher formal education also tend to pay more attention to news and information programmes and less to entertainment programmes than the less educated. In addition, they seem to make use of more sources of information. In a study on SES and smoking, Millar (1996) found that lower SES groups reported fewer sources of information about smoking and were less likely to report printed information sources than higher SES groups. Similar results were reported by Finnegan *et al.* (1993) in relation to information about heart disease. They found that groups with lower formal education report fewer sources of information than groups with higher formal education. Thus we discern a tendency: 'to those who have (information), to those will be given'. Differences are also found in relation to the impact of mass media information. This phenomenon is referred to as the 'knowledge gap' (Tichenor *et al.*, 1970). Both more highly and more lowly educated people benefit from mass media information in terms of knowledge, but the more highly educated benefit more. Hence, the gap is enlarged by the mass media. An increasing number of attempts have been made to reach less educated target groups by 'sandwiching' information programmes between two popular entertainment programmes. The entertainment-education approach seems to be promising in this regard.

6.2 Interpersonal methods

Most of the conventional mass media are characterised by a one-sided flow of information. There is no direct contact between the sender and the receiver and, consequently, there is no direct feedback about whether or not the receiver sees the message and will use that information in any way. In contrast, direct feedback is a major advantage of interpersonal communication, especially in situations where there is direct contact between the communication parties, i.e. non-mediated communications. The sender can observe the receiver, at least to some extent, and sender and receiver can easily change roles. In this section we start with the most direct interaction method, that is, one-to-one communication, or, as we call it, dialogue. Thereafter we discuss lectures, and proceed via demonstrations to small group methods.

6.2.1 Dialogue

The most personalised communication method is dialogue, also referred to as mutual discussion, counselling, or personal instruction. In health communication, dialogue is probably the method most widely used. Consider the work of general practitioners, dentists, paediatricians, dieticians, psychiatrists, nurses, and physiotherapists. Dialogue has several advantages over less personalised methods. It gives a health professional the opportunity to get to know the person well, and to get first hand information on problems and their possible causes. Possibilities for, and constraints on, solving problems as perceived by the client are easily accessible and can be placed in the specific context of the client. Dialogue is a more effective instrument in stimulating people to change behaviour than more general information. Russell *et al.* (1987) found that even short inquiries and discussions between doctors and patients about smoking results in an increased cessation rate of about five per cent compared with general information giving. Clearly, the credibility of one's own physician or dietician is important, but the direct link with one's personal situation can have a particularly powerful impact. Dialogue offers a good opportunity for tailoring, that is, information and instruction that is adjusted to the unique problem of the person in question (see section 4.1.4). Naturally, dialogue has disadvantages too. It is inefficient in that its reach is small, and the cost per person reached is high. Furthermore, often only those clients who are aware of having a problem (usually when the problem is well advanced and has caused some difficulty) will initiate mutual discussion. People generally will not consult a dietician before there is a felt need to change dietary habits.

Various models of dialogue have been developed. We will consider three of these models in more detail: the diagnosis-prescription model, the counselling model, and the participation model.

- The *diagnosis-prescription model* originates from the traditional doctor-patient relationship and is based on what we called the medical approach in section 2.2. It is a typical, expert-led method, where the expert asks a series of questions. Based on the answers, the expert diagnoses the nature of the problem and its possible causes, and gives prescriptions and advice. Clients merely have a passive role. This model has been, and still is, very popular, especially in patient education. It should be realised, however, that little learning takes place, since the client does not actively contribute to the diagnosis of the problem, or to finding possible solutions. The model is useful if the parties involved feel that the expert indeed has the appropriate expertise, if both parties feel comfortable with it and agree about the goals to be achieved, and if the client just wants to receive advice. However, research has shown that this method is unsuitable for more complicated problems - problems in which emotions play an important role, or problems that cannot be solved in the short term.
- The *counselling model* has been developed by Rogers (1962), for psychotherapeutic purposes. Rogers considers that people are prone to many psychiatric problems if their self-image does not fit the way others react to them. They dare not assimilate these reactions into their own self-image, but they can be helped with this problem through the use of non-directive discussion techniques. It is a client-centred approach, emphasising the actual feelings and experiences of the client and focusing on creating an encouraging atmosphere. The client determines the topics discussed, and the client's feelings and interpretations are the point of departure. The counsellor does not act like an expert, but listens to the client, asks questions, and helps clients to clarify and structure their feelings and needs as well as the possibilities for addressing these problems. Counsellors (e.g. health professionals) refrain from giving their own views, but show that they understand and accept what clients say

about their feelings by repeating them in their own words. This is called 'reflection' or 'mirroring'. The counselling approach is especially useful for problems in which emotions play an important role (for example, coping with a chronic disease), or problems that cannot be solved in the short term (for example, changes in lifestyle).

- *The participation model* reflects dialogue situations in which both the expert and the client play an active role in diagnosis of problems, in the analysis of possible causes, and in problem solving. The professional contributes expertise only if the client appears to need it, and the client makes decisions where possible. As a rule, discussion will begin along counselling lines in order to get a clear picture of the client's goals and of why he or she thinks he or she has not yet achieved these goals. This may result in a redefinition of the problem. In the next phase, the client contributes factual information and, if necessary, the professional adds to it. This allows them to see which alternative solutions are possible and what results can be expected from each of these alternatives. If it appears to be impossible to reach the goals that have initially been set, these goals must be adapted to the possibilities. When a choice is being made among the alternatives, discussion will again be more in the form of counselling, because the client is responsible for the choice. The model is very useful for complex problems, or problems that cannot be solved in the short term.

Which model is chosen will depend on the extent to which relevant knowledge lies with the expert, with the client, or with both, and on who is considered to have the right to decide about goals to be achieved. If a patient has a broken leg, nearly all the knowledge about how to cure this problem may lie with the doctor. However, if the doctor has told a patient that he is likely to die from cancer within a few months, counselling is perhaps the best way to discover how he can adjust his life to this information. The participation model fits better with the current approach in health education and health promotion than the diagnosis-description model. Also, counselling and participatory approaches often seem to be more effective. For instance, based on a review of medical research literature, DiNicolla and DiMatteo (1984) conclude that patient compliance is usually very low if a therapy is based on this diagnosis-prescription model. For example, as many as half of the patients with active illnesses fail to take the medications prescribed by physicians at medical clinics. Even people with acute and painful illnesses, like gastrointestinal ulcers, ignore the prescribed regimen. Among the possible causes of non-compliance are failure of the physician to make the patient clearly understand the instructions, failure to adapt the therapy to the everyday-life situation of the patient, and a lack of patient participation in decisions about the therapy. These problems can be overcome more adequately when counselling or participatory methods are used.

6.2.2 Lectures

Lectures are in fact the oldest means of transferring information. Despite their relatively high cost per capita in comparison with the mass media, lectures have some specific advantages. Firstly, the speaker can modify the content of the talk to meet the specific needs and interests of the audience as well as their level of education. The speaker can take account of audience response during the talk (feedback) and modify his or her approach accordingly. Secondly, the audience gets to know the speaker better and receives a clearer impression of his or her feelings about the subject through gestures and facial expressions. Thirdly, lectures usually provide an opportunity for the audience to ask questions and discuss issues in greater depth. The disadvantage with lectures is that the spoken word is usually forgotten more easily than the written word. It is difficult to maintain an audience's attention on the subject of a talk for much longer than 15 minutes, unless the speaker is extremely dynamic and interesting. People's thoughts tend to wander to other unrelated issues. Written materials can be re-read if something is not immediately clear, but a listener may quickly lose the thread or forget the main points in a talk. Lectures are also poor methods for teaching how to apply information. To achieve this objective, lectures must be combined with discussions and practical demonstrations. Information is more likely to be remembered and acted upon in the future if the audience is stimulated into actively thinking about the issues being discussed. Hence it is good practice to combine lectures with other techniques. Lectures are often followed by a question-and-answer session, which allows the listeners to clarify their understanding. A lecture followed by a discussion may be used to focus public attention on a problem. For example, a speaker may give little information during the talk, but may ask many questions. These questions then become the topics for discussion following the talk. In the case of larger groups, it is preferable to divide the audience into small discussion groups so that all group members have the opportunity to present their views. Information discussed in the small groups may then be summarised in a plenary session in which the whole audience participates. Reserving sufficient time for discussion is crucial for the stimulation of active learning.

6.2.3 Demonstrations

A demonstration is a performance-oriented method that stimulates the audience to try out innovations themselves. Demonstrations are based on the idea that people can learn a lot from their own experience, but also from observing the experience of their peers (i.e. vicarious learning; see section 3.2.2). It is a helpful method for skill building (psychomotor) activities, but also for increasing feelings of self-efficacy. Demonstrations provide opportunities to supply information about procedures, give explanations of methods, and enable experimentation with advised methods. They can show causes of problems and possible solutions without complicated technical details. Demonstrations can be used to show *results* of certain actions, for example the results of a weight-loss programme. Moreover, they can be used to show *methods*. Examples are: classes in which people learn how to prepare low-fat meals, courses in which parents learn how to play with their children, instruction programmes for breast self-examination, teeth-brushing lessons for children, or courses for teachers on how to act if a student suffers an epilepsy seizure. Demonstrations may be conducted in individual settings as well as in groups.

6.2.4 Group methods

Group methods are used for many different purposes in different societies. Committee meetings are used at a political level to achieve consensus or unanimous decisions. In health promotion, group methods may be used to involve people in community coalitions (see Chapter 7). Similar to one-to-one dialogue, in health education, group methods are used to help people identify and find solutions to their problems. Group methods have an advantage over the mass media because of the possibility of obtaining direct feedback about how information is perceived. This facilitates the reduction of misunderstandings that may develop between the communicator and the receiver. Moreover, and additional to dialogue, group methods stimulate interaction between the participants. This interaction provides the opportunity for participants to exchange useful experiences. However, per capita costs of group methods tend to be much higher than for mass media. Group methods can take many different forms. Two of these have become increasingly popular in health education and health promotion: the peer-group method and self-help groups.

The central feature of *peer groups* is that the 'educator' and the 'educated' are members of the same (social) group. It is designed to be 'by-and-for' the group involved. For instance, adults educating adults about preventive sexual behaviour, asthma patients educating asthma patients about self-management, the elderly educating the elderly about healthy nutrition. Peer education has been applied in a variety of settings, such as schools and community centres, and related to a variety of issues, such as the reduction of smoking among adults (e.g. Telch *et al.*, 1990), substance misuse (Klepp *et al.*, 1986), sex education (e.g. Phelps *et al.*, 1994), HIV prevention (e.g. Kelly *et al.*, 1991), and ethnic-specific diabetes education (e.g. Voorham, 2003). Programmes such as Mothers Inform Mothers, in which experienced mothers provide parenting support for first-time mothers (Hanrahan *et al.*, 1997), are also based on the concept of peer education. Evaluation of 'community mother programmes' provides evidence that peer education is also beneficial to those involved in providing it (Molloy, 1997). It is assumed that peers are more successful than professionals in passing on information, because people can identify with their peers. In line with this, it is claimed that peer education can be used to educate those who are hard to reach through conventional methods. Moreover, it is claimed that peer educators act as positive role models (for an overview of claims on the working of peer education, we refer to Turner & Shepherd, 1999).

Another popular method is that of *self-help groups*. Self-help groups are organised around a common problem of its participants and characterised by little or no involvement of professional helpers. At the core of self-help groups lies the notion that members participating in these groups benefit from sharing their experiences, strengths and hopes and thereby come closer to solving their problems (Welch-Cline,

1999). Interacting with other people with comparable or even greater problems than one's own can reduce the sense of isolation, increase feelings of receiving support, and provide a variety of useful coping approaches (Mechanic, 1999). Alcoholics Anonymous (AA) is probably the best-known example, but self-help groups cover a broad range of issues relating to health and illness. In a survey of 232 members from 65 disease-related self-help groups, Trojan (1989) found self-reported benefits in different areas of life of the patients. Here, we give only a few examples. In relation to disease and wellbeing, 70 per cent of the participants reported a reduction in emotional stress, and 62 per cent a reduction in fear of a disease crisis. In addition, 92 per cent reported having learned new behaviour, 61 per cent took up more socialising activities, and 95 per cent reported more rational utilisation of medication. Positive results from self-help groups have been found for groups of psychiatric patients, patients with chronic disease, cancer patients, HIV/AIDS infected persons, people with disabilities, relatives of the chronically ill, and parents of young drug abusers.

6.2.5 Effects of small group methods

For group methods to be effective, group size is important. When the group is too small there will be insufficient input for discussion and, if the group is too large, several participants will refrain from taking part in the discussion. Generally it is recommended that a group size be chosen of between five and fifteen participants. Experts can play different roles in a group. In lectures for example, they are usually the expert source of information, and hence perceived to be above their audience in status. However, in discussion groups they participate as group members who join all other members in solving problems. In peer groups and self-help groups they have only a 'background function'. What can be achieved with group methods?

Increasing knowledge: Small group methods assist the process of transferring knowledge from an expert to the group, although the printed word and audiovisual material, as well as lectures, are cheaper, more structured and usually more effective for this purpose. However, group discussion helps people assimilate knowledge by giving the participants an opportunity to ask questions, to relate the new information to what they already know, and, if necessary, to revise their views. Then if lingering doubts remain, they can discuss them with the other participants and/or with the discussion leader. Expert-led group discussions do not necessarily contain the most useful knowledge. As mentioned under the sections on peer groups and self-help groups, other group members may have better or more valuable information to contribute. A diabetic patient may want to hear from a doctor about the nature and consequences of the disease, but fellow discussion group members may be of more use in providing information about how to cope with this disease in everyday life.

Change in frame of reference: Small group methods can fulfil several functions in relation to change in frame of reference. Firstly, they can help in *creating awareness of problems and feelings.* People are inclined to evade problems if forced to choose between two alternatives, both of which have unpleasant consequences. Furthermore, people are often only partially aware of their feelings. Group discussion can help to eliminate these constraints on decision making by increasing the awareness of problems and of feelings. It is sometimes easier to acknowledge one's feelings in a group where other members openly discuss their own feelings too. This function of group methods is often used in counselling programmes involving, for example, marital problems, but also in self-help groups of, for example, HIV-infected persons, cancer patients, or the parents of children with disabilities. Secondly, group methods can help to arrive at *concrete formulations of problems.* The more clearly a problem can be defined, the more likely it is a solution will be found. Group discussions can help to specify problems clearly and in more detail. Thirdly, group discussion can help participants to *form an opinion* about a specific issue or new development. Formation of 'sound' opinions results from mutual testing of ideas among group members. This does not necessarily mean that opinions are uniform, but it does ensure they have been considered more carefully. Fourthly, they can lead to a *change in norms.* In Chapter 3 we discussed the important influence of social norms on individual behaviour. These norms do not change if an outsider, e.g. a health communicator, says they are old fashioned. Consider what we said in section 5.3.2 about the difficulty of realising changes in attitudes that makes the receiver a deviant in his or her own social environment. However, if the group itself concludes that they should change attitudes and norms, they indeed do change. Group discussion can lead to a change in norms, especially if various participants have already accepted the change but incorrectly believe that their fellow group members still adhere to the 'old' viewpoint.

Behaviour change: Group methods can also lead to behaviour change. Lewin (1953) demonstrated the important role of group discussion in *individual decision making* in a series of famous experiments. He compared the effects of group discussion and individual advice when mothers were being taught to give their babies cod liver oil. One group of mothers, about to leave hospital, held group discussions about the best ways to feed their babies and took a group decision that each should give them cod liver oil. Another group received individual advice on the same topic. Four weeks later, 85 per cent of group discussion participants had given cod liver oil, compared with 55 per cent of those given individual advice. According to Lewin, the change of group norms is an important link in the change process. We also wish to refer to section 3.7.1, where we have seen that, especially in new and unknown situations, group members possess informational social influence: individuals tend to accept such group decisions and they internalise these decisions.

Collective decisions: Group discussion leads to a *collective decision* in many committees. Group discussion can have an important role in helping people become aware of their collective interests and in deciding how they can best protect these interests. For example, dirty playgrounds for children in a neighbourhood often start to get dirty because a few leave waste in such an area, prompting others to do the same. Since playgrounds are public places, no one feels personally responsible for cleaning up. Discussion groups are valuable tools for mobilising community action to overcome such problems. Doubts may linger about whether or not we have made the right choice between alternatives, especially when the choice is important and we have hesitated to make a decision. For example, someone who has decided to follow a diet to lose weight, but in putting it into practice is faced with problems such as trying to resist offered cakes, may feel a strong need to discuss with others who have made similar decisions whether or not they have made the right choice, and to look for solutions to any adjustment difficulties. In these situations, group discussion helps to reduce uncertainty. These discussions generally strengthen a person's decision to implement the choice already made, thus leading to a confirmation of the choice. We can gain some further insight into the function of group methods by comparing its advantages and disadvantages with lectures. This is summarised in Table 6.1.

Table 6.1 Advantages and disadvantages of group methods compared with lectures.

Advantages	Disadvantages
Participants discuss more aspects than the change agent does on his or her own.	The transfer of information takes more time.
Participants are better judges than the change agent whether possible solutions are practical.	Problems are discussed less systematically than in a lecture.
In a group discussion there is a strong tie with daily practice that is not usually present in a lecture.	There is a danger that some participants will 'ride their hobby horses' or dominate discussion.
Language used in discussion is more familiar to participants.	A good discussion assumes participants have at least minimal knowledge.
Participants can ask questions, present opposing ideas, which improve assimilation of what is said.	There is a chance that incorrect information given by one group member will not be corrected.
Group discussions stimulate participants' own activities much more than lectures.	Group discussions require a discussion leader who can handle unexpected problems that may arise.
Participants have opportunity to discover unknown aspects of a problem. This increases the probability that they adopt solutions discussed by the group.	The socio-emotional climate has a great influence on the effects of group discussions. It is not always easy to influence this climate in a positive way.
Participants will generally be more interested, . because they can exert influence on the choice of problems to be discussed.	Group discussions require a certain degree of homogeneity in the group.
Group discussions can have a significant effect on transfer of information and on decision-making.	For discussions, group size should not exceed 15 participants; lectures can be held for much larger groups.
Group norms can be considered at a group discussion, and changed by the group, if necessary.	
Discussion leaders learn more about knowledge levels, experiences, and problems of group members than speakers.	
	Cost per person reached is high.

6.3 Hybrid media

Especially since the early 1990s a new group of media, mostly based on computer technology (ICT), has become popular, the so-called hybrid media. Hybrid media combine the potentials offered by the mass media and by interpersonal communication, in that they potentially reach large numbers of people in many different locations, but at the same time support a level of interactivity that is higher than with conventional mass media (Leeuwis & van den Ban, 2004). Examples are CD-ROM (Compact Disc-Read Only Memory), CD-i (Compact Disc-interactive), DVD (optical disc storage; 'digital video disc') and electronic conferencing systems. As the costs involved in using such technologies are declining rapidly (Shapiro & Varian, 1999; World Bank, 1998), their potential for communicative interventions is increasing. Hybrid media have potential for health communication, and indeed are increasingly used in our field. Computerised technology makes it possible to reach large audiences, whilst at the same time it can adjust to the specific needs of a small audience and even to the individual. The interactive media in particular make personalisation possible. In the early 1990s there was a large variety of 'new media', and for each of these the user needed to have special software and hardware in order to use them. Today, most of these systems have become accessible and/or available on one electronic platform: the Internet (see Leeuwis & van den Ban, 2004). With the Internet, several new modalities of information transfer emerged, such as the World Wide Web, electronic mail, news groups and chat rooms. We will discuss some of these applications, meant to reach large audiences, small groups, and applications for tailor-made assistance.

World Wide Web: Many organisations and individuals nowadays have a website. A website is essentially an advanced multi-channel (textual, auditive, visual) brochure that can be opened at a specific electronic address, i.e. a computer that is connected to a worldwide computer network. The brochure can contain just text pages, but can also use animations, pictures, video clips, voices, sound or music (Leeuwis & van den Ban, 2004). Health organisations increasingly provide information through their website about a broad area of health-related topics. Information can be found, for example, about specific diseases and medical problems (e.g. the 'net doctor'), about nutrition and healthy diets, alcohol and drug abuse, sexually transmittable diseases, physical exercise and fitness, depression and anxiety, stress, mental health issues, but also about the organisations themselves (e.g. their mission, services and deliverables). And, indeed, a growing number of people all over the world turn to the Internet (*Cyber Atlas*, 2003), to look for health information also (*cf.* Rice & Katz, 2001). Surveys from Pew Internet and American Life (2003) show that 80 per cent of US adult Internet users have searched for information on health issues. It should be realised, however, that people 'visiting' the website do not all have the same information needs. It is assumed that they search and sift through the information and select that information which is relevant to their personal needs.

Online support groups: Coinciding with the increased popularity of the Internet has been the growing popularity of 'virtual communities'. These are Internet platforms on which a large variety of people come together in groups that are devoted to a range of topics. In a sense, they are comparable to chat rooms, but in virtual communities the communicating partners need not be active on the Internet at the same time. A specific type of such virtual community is the online support group. A survey from Pew Internet and American Life (2003) reveals that Internet users increasingly visit disease-specific support sites to discuss health issues. Support groups can be found on a broad spectrum of health-related topics, such as AIDS, alcohol and drug addictions, different types of cancer, cerebral palsy, chronic fatigue syndrome, diabetes, eating disorders, people with disabilities, suicide, heart disease or depression. The online support groups in fact work in a similar way to what we previously called the self-help groups (*cf.* Lamerichs, 2003).

Computer tailoring: In section 6.2.1 we discussed the topic of tailoring of information and of change strategies, intended to reach one person. Tailoring is also possible by using interactive technology, i.e. computer tailoring. In computer tailoring, the expertise of one or more counsellors is translated into a series of 'if then' statements and as such documented in an expert system. After this system has been developed, it can be applied and distributed relatively independently of the experts (Brug *et al.*, 2003). The process of computer tailoring attempts to mimic the process of personal counselling. People are surveyed or interviewed, and the results are keyed or automatically scanned into a data file. The tailoring expert system analyses these data and links them with a feedback and advice source, which is a message library or archive that contains appropriate feedback and advice for each survey response (Brug *et al.*, 2003:1030S). Although the effects of computer tailoring have mainly been studied in relation to nutrition behaviours, research shows that automated individual feedback is more effective than general information (*cf.* Brug *et al.*, 2003; Oenema *et al.*, 2001). A great advantage of computer tailoring is that it makes personalisation applicable to large groups of people, and at relatively low cost compared to personal counselling.

As mentioned before, hybrid media combine aspects of both the mass media and interpersonal forms of communication. Accordingly, hybrid media share the advantages and disadvantages of these forms of communication. We do not wish to discuss these aspects extensively, but summarise them in Table 6.2.

6.4 Mass media and interpersonal methods in health communication

Mass media and interpersonal methods each have their specific characteristics. Table 6.3 provides a comparison between these methods, by listing some of the central features of each. This comparison can help to develop insight into the advantages and disadvantages of the different methods. As we argued in the previous section, hybrid media resemble basic forms of mass media in some respects, and interpersonal communication in others. We therefore do not include hybrid media explicitly in the overview. For the sake of brevity, we also ignore differences between the various mass media and between the different interpersonal methods. Also, we ignore the influence of mass media devices when used in conjunction with interpersonal communication.

It is clear from what we have already discussed that each method has its own advantages and disadvantages. Hence there is not much sense in asking which method is the best. One always has to consider what function each method can fulfil in health communication. It is not uncommon for health communicators to continue using one particular educational approach simply because it has worked in previous situations, or because they are familiar with it. In choosing a specific

Table 6.2 Potential qualities of hybrid media in comparison with those of mass media and interpersonal communication.

Potential functional quality	Resemblance to mass media or interpersonal forms	Clarification
Audience reached	Like mass media	• Potentially a world-wide audience (if access exists; this varies greatly across countries and social strata) • Less direct spin-offs than, for example, television as messages often are not received in groups
Mobilising attention	Less than other media	• Hybrid media tend to be less visible in everyday life • Difficult to find relevant information due to overload
Specificity/ tailor made/ active learning	In between	• Some degree of specificity is possible in case of (prestructured) man-computer interaction • Less intensive exchange in case of man-man interaction
Relational support	Like mass media	• Difficult to establish relationships of trust due to limited social presence
Insight in audience	In between	• Audiences can respond to messages through e-mail • Users' way of using hybrid media can be registered
Speed/ actuality	Faster than mass media	• News and actualities are often available on the internet before they are broadcast by radio/television • Websites/programmes can be centrally updated, and be immediately available to everyone
Time flexibility	Like written mass media	• Internet can be consulted whenever it suits the user
Spatial flexibility	Often like audio-visual mass media	• Equipment, electricity and network cess are often tied to locations (but mobile equipment is spreading)
Storage capacity	Like written mass media	• A message received can be stored on a computer or printed, and accessed again if needed
External/ internal skills	Like mass media	• A simple website can be built easily by internal staff, but advanced applications require special skills
Dependence on others	Much less than mass media	• With the internet everybody has in principle his or her own broadcasting station and editorial board
Cost per person	Mostly in between	• Development and maintenance costs of hybrid media can be rather high

Source: Leeuwis & van den Ban (2004: 204).

Table 6.3 Differences between mass media and interpersonal communication.

Characteristic	Interpersonal channels	Mass media channe
Message flow	Tends to be two-way	Tends to be one-way
Communication context	Face-to-face	Interposed
Amount of feedback readily available	High	Low
Ability to overcome selective processes	High	Low
Speed to large audiences	Relatively slow	Relatively rapid
Possibility to adjust message to audience	Large	Small
Cost per person reached	High	Low
Possibility for audience to ignore	Low	High
Same message to all receivers	No	Yes
Who gives information	Everybody	Expert or power hold
Possible effect	Attitude formation and change	Knowledge change

Adapted from Rogers, E .M. and Shoemaker, F. F. (1971: 253).

method or a combination of methods, we have to be mindful of the objectives we want to achieve, the complexity of the behaviour or of the health problem addressed, the complexity of the situation, and the stage of change in which the targets are.

In Table 6.4 we integrate the stages of change, the requirements to enable change in each stage, and the strategies and methods that relate to that. With health communication, we usually try to achieve objectives in which time plays an important role. Objectives relating to positive changes in behaviour can generally only be achieved in the long term. They require regular and multiple inputs of information and action (Koelen *et al.*, 2001). There may be an optimum method for each purpose or function to be fulfilled, but there is no best method for all circumstances. It is therefore recommended that different methods be purposely integrated into one programme, so that they reinforce each other. Research has shown that different information sources are used at the beginning and the end of the rather lengthy process of adopting an innovation. The mass media can be very influential at the beginning of the change process (e.g. making people aware, increasing knowledge, shaping or changing opinions). The mass media are relatively ineffective in changing behaviour. Interpersonal methods like

Table 6.4 Communication methods related to stages of change.

Stage of change	Requirement	Strategy	Methods
Precontemplation • Awareness • Attention	• exposure to communication • paying attention • becoming interested	Transfer of information (from outside)	Publications and recommendations in mass media, internet, lectures, leaflets, directive dialogue
Contemplation • Knowledge • Pros and cons	• comprehension • information search and retrieval		
Preparation • Intention • Decision	• attitude change • subjective norms/ social influence • self-efficacy/skill acquisition • decision to change	Learning by experience (information from inside)	Group discussions, non-directive dialogue, tailor-made ICT, certain types of films
Action • Implementation	• behaving in accordance with decision	Exercise in skills	Methods which encourage action, such as training, demonstration, modelling by films, small groups
Maintenance • Continued adoption	• reinforcement • consolidation	Confirmation of choice	Providing feedback through publications and recommendations in mass media, lectures, leaflets, tailor-made ICT

demonstrations and small group discussions are more influential in the 'middle range'. At the end of the change process, the mass media can again be influential because they provide information about how the intention to change can be implemented, for example, which food is low in cholesterol. Mass media can also be influential for the purpose of providing feedback (confirmation).

Sometimes different methods will be used at the same time - for example, a lecture supported by audiovisual aids. Sometimes they will be used in succession, as when written materials are used to prepare participants for a group discussion, or when written materials are given out after a demonstration to provide the possibility of re-reading. In fact, a multimedia approach is important not only in performing each vital function in the communication process, but also in performing it through the most suitable medium. Advertising research has shown that a person receiving the same message through different media will pay more attention because he or she recognises something familiar from another context.

When planning combinations of media we should think not only of large, well-organised campaigns, but also of using audiovisual aids to support lectures and group discussions. In this context we refer to devices such as whiteboards, flipcharts, overhead and video projectors, photographs, drawings, graphs, maps, slides, film, radio, television, sound and videotapes, CD-ROMs, and programmed learning terminals.

6.5 Chapter summary

In this chapter we have spelled out strengths and weaknesses of different communication methods. We made it clear that advantages and disadvantages depend not only on the specific method used, but also on the objectives to be achieved, the complexity of the behaviour, and on the stage of change in which the target group is at the time. Instead of a summary, we refer to Table 6.5, which reviews some of the

Table 6.5 Functions, advantages and disadvantages of different communication methods.

Medium suitable for:	Mass media	Lectures	Demonstration	Group discussions	Dialogue
Creating awareness of innovations	XXX	X	XX	0	0
Creating awareness of individual problems	0	X	XX	XXX	XXX
Knowledge transfer	XXX	XX	XX	X	XX
Behavioural change	0	0	XX	XXX	XX
Using others' knowledge	0	0	X	XXX	X
Activating learning processes	0	0	X	XXX	XX
Adjustment to personal problems	0	0	X	XX	XXX
Cost per person reached*	X	XX	XX	XXX	XXXX

0= unsuitable. The number of crosses indicates suitability, except where marked with an asterisk which indicates the level of abstraction advantages and disadvantages of the methods discussed. It should be noted that, in the table, the nature of the audience and the nature of the message receive only limited treatment. Furthermore, many of the points outlined in the table are based on impressions rather than on established research results.

7. Community participation and intersectoral collaboration

In the previous chapter we discussed communication methods that are useful for the dissemination of information about health issues. The focus was very much on informing and influencing individual receivers, thus on health education. In this chapter we put our emphasis on the broader perspective of health promotion. As addressed earlier, a central approach in health promotion is that of community action. The point of departure is people's everyday lives. This means that health promotion has to take place in those places where people live, work, and play. In doing so, it aims at individual behaviour and lifestyle, but considers the socio-economic and environmental conditions in which behaviour takes place as important prerequisites for healthy lifestyles. Hence, the improvement of conditions that affect people's health status is an essential strategy for the facilitation of health-sustaining lifestyles. Health promotion is not imposed on people, but aims to work together with people, in the setting of their everyday lives. Consequently, the participation of the target population is considered essential. Health promotion eventually strives for empowerment of communities and people living in these communities. Moreover, as we spelled out in previous chapters, the promotion of health is a matter of concern for a broad spectrum of sectors and organisations. It benefits from the collaborative action of professionals and non-professionals from the health sector, and all other sectors that affect health in its broadest sense.

Community action is thus governed by concepts of intersectoral collaboration and community participation. But what is meant by it? And why is it so important? Does it work? Is it as easy as words would have us believe? These questions will be addressed in this chapter. Firstly we will discuss and define the concepts of community, community participation and intersectoral collaboration. Since community participation and intersectoral collaboration are expected to lead to empowerment, we will also elaborate to some extent on this concept. We then suggest how community action can be organised, and pay attention to the forces that might inhibit or facilitate such action.

7.1 Defining communities

The concept of 'community' is often used in health promotion literature, either in scientific articles, working papers, or in national and international policy documents. This indicates that there is a general understanding of the concept. Nothing could be less true however. Ashton (1988:183), for example, refers to an article that mentions that there are at least 90 definitions of 'community' in sociology. Tones and Tilford (1994) refer to a paper of Hubley (1985) who found 94 definitions. Among these numerous definitions, two broad lines can be distinguished, that is: (1) definitions in terms of geographical area, and (2) definitions in terms of shared characteristics.

The Oxford dictionary defines community in geographical terms as: 'the people living in one place, district or country, considered as a whole'. In health literature, such geographical definitions are also used, for example Agudelo's (1983) definition 'a group of people living in a particular area, sharing values, cultural patterns and social problems'. Rifkin *et al.* (2000) argue that such definitions reflect the views of epidemiologists who look for 'target groups at risk' within geographical areas on which to focus interventions. Definitions in terms of shared characteristics refer to the existence of potential resources such as people's skills and knowledge in social networks. In this way, communities are seen as groups of people with common perceptions of needs, interest, and priorities, who can express their relationships without difficulty through communication. In the WHO Health Promotion Glossary (Nutbeam, 1998:5), features of both lines of definition are combined. Community is defined as: 'a specific group of people, often living in a defined geographical area, who share a common culture, values and norms, and are arranged in a social structure according to relationships which the community has developed over a period of time. Members of a community gain their personal and social identity by sharing common beliefs, values and norms, which have been developed by the community in the past and may be modified in the future. They exhibit some awareness of their identity as a group, and share common needs and a commitment to meeting them.'

In our opinion, we have to be cautious when using the geographical dimension, because geography is often a weak factor in defining people's common interests. People living in the same area, working in the same factory, or in the same school, do not necessarily have the same views or interests. Also, people do not belong to one but to a range of communities, varying from, for example, family, sports club, school, and workplace, to church. Moreover, communities are not static, but dynamic. Communities change as members move away and new ones move in. In addition, new (virtual) communities come into being through the increasing possibilities and actual use of modern communication systems like the Internet and the World Wide Web, transcending geographical boundaries and localities. This indicates that the non-geographic dimensions such as affinity, common goals, shared interests, and social interaction are equally, or even more, important. A definition which takes into account most of these remarks has been formulated by Laverack and Labonte (2000:258; also see section 4.2.4), that is: 'communities are organised groups that are important enough to their individual members, who identify themselves, in part, by that group membership'.

Communities, however, are not only a compilation of people. They also include social institutions, which can be communities in their own right. For example, in a geographic community such as a residential area, we may find social institutions such as schools, shops and restaurants, churches, health centres, business and work facilities, recreational areas, coalitions, and influence networks. In addition, communities include social control components, such as legislation, formal and informal rules, and value and norm systems. All these components have special relevance in relation to community organisation. Given the complexity, it is not surprising that so many definitions exist. It should be realised that communities are often defined by outsiders, for example by professionals who want to impose a specific intervention on that community. In our opinion, a community only exists if its members feel themselves to be (a part of) that community. It is therefore important to discuss the meaning of 'community' with the people involved, and it should be defined in light of the target group, the institutions, and the locality with which its members identify.

Based on the previous discussion, we define communities as *groups of people who identify themselves by their group membership, sharing a common interest, common social institutions and common social control components.*

7.2 Community participation

Just as there are many definitions of community, community participation has also been defined in a number of different ways. Three common characteristics are found in these definitions. Firstly, the definitions refer to involvement of *individual* community members. This is important, because it is unrealistic to expect total community participation. Communities can be large, and this makes it practically impossible to involve all members. In these situations, broad participation through representation should be sought; but even if a community is relatively small, this is unrealistic. Consider, for example, what was said about adopter categories in Chapter 4. Secondly, most definitions consider community participation to be a *process*, which means that it consists of interactions and feedback. It has to develop over time. Thirdly, they include phrases such as 'involvement in problem analysis, needs assessment and setting priorities', 'involvement in development, implementation and evaluation of health promoting activities', and 'taking part in decision making at all levels'. Here we use the following definition: *community participation is a process whereby community members take part in the identification of their needs, setting priorities, identifying and obtaining means to meet those priorities, including the development, implementation and evaluation of those means in terms of their outcomes*. It should be noted that this definition can apply not only to geographical areas, like certain parts of a city, but also to settings such as schools, workplaces, hospitals or prisons.

7.3 Intersectoral collaboration

Determinants of health are intertwined in almost all sectors of society. Hence, improving individual and community health is not the responsibility of the health sector alone, but a collective responsibility. Intersectoral collaboration is one of the guiding principles adopted at the International Conference on Primary Health Care for achieving health goals (WHO, 1978). The notion underlying this principle is that, in order to achieve satisfactory levels of health, the health sector should work together with other sectors that contribute to (influence) health. These sectors could be, for example, environment, transport, industry, employment, agriculture, animal husbandry, food industry, education, housing, public works and communication. It can be collaboration between the public sphere, the private sphere, the voluntary sphere and individuals. Intersectoral collaboration can be defined as 'a recognised relationship between (parts of) different sectors of society, which has been formed to take action on an issue to achieve health outcomes in a way which is more effective, efficient or sustainable than might be achieved by the health sector acting alone' (*cf.* Nutbeam, 1998:14).

Intersectoral action is expected to bring about changes in at least two directions. It should lead to the improvement of determinants of health and thereby of the health of individuals and communities. In addition, it should increase the awareness of the health consequences involved in policy decisions and organisational practice, within and among different sectors. The complexity of this latter aim can be illustrated by the example of the food production system. The handling of products in each part of the chain, from primary production to food preparation in household kitchens, includes health-related issues, such as pesticide use in primary production, additives in industry, and hygiene in households. The food chain thus involves a wide range of people and organisations, including the farmer and his family, the primary production supply industry (e.g. seed, pesticides), the food processing industry, transport, the wholesale trade, supermarkets and the consumer, and many more. They all have different, often conflicting, interests and perspectives. Decisions in each part of the chain have consequences for the outcomes in the other parts. These include economic, personal and social consequences, but also environmental and health consequences, and their interrelationships. The example shows the need to reconcile and negotiate between different interests and perspectives. Intersectoral action creates opportunities for exchanging values, expertise, skills and resources. It has the potential for synergy, where the whole is equal to more than the sum of its parts. It is expected that intersectoral action will eventually lead to a movement in the direction of healthy public policy, that is, a policy that is characterised by a concern for health and equity in all areas of policy, and by accountability for the health impact.

7.4 Empowerment

Intersectoral collaboration and community participation are considered to be the key strategies leading to empowerment. But what does empowerment actually mean? According to the Oxford dictionary, to empower someone means 'to give power or authority to act'. In health promotion, the term empowerment is considered to be the process through which people gain greater control over decisions and actions affecting their health (Nutbeam, 1998). Here we clearly see the resemblance to the definition of health promotion, i.e. the process of enabling people to increase control over, and to improve, their health. Yet, in spite of extensive research and several programmes that aim at empowerment, there is still no clearly measurable operationalisation of the concept. Rappaport (1985; 1987) argues that it is difficult to define empowerment in terms of outcomes, because it includes psychological and political components, and it will look different in its manifest content for different people, organisations and settings. Empowerment is easy to recognise when it happens, but the absence of empowerment is also easy to recognise: powerlessness, learned helplessness and alienation are all terms that reflect the absence of empowerment. Rissel (1994) proposes making a distinction between psychological empowerment and community empowerment. *Psychological empowerment* refers to a *subjective feeling* of greater control over one's own life experienced by an individual following active memberships in groups or organisations, and it may occur without participation in collective political action. It is assessed with the individual as a unit of analysis (Bracht *et al.*, 1999). Psychological empowerment relates to such concepts as perceived self-efficacy, internal locus of control, self-acceptance and self-confidence. *Community empowerment* reflects a state of communities or subgroups within communities. According to Rissel (1994), it includes a raised level of psychological empowerment among its members, a political action component in which members have actively participated, and the achievement of some redistribution of resources or decision making favourable to the community group in question.

The definitions so far refer to a 'state', or to a feeling. But psychological and community empowerment are the result of a *process* of personal development, participation and social action. This is also reflected in Wallerstein's (1992:198) definition of community empowerment, that is, 'a social action process that promotes participation of people, organisations, and communities towards the goals of increased individual and community control, political efficacy, improved quality of community life, and social justice'. Participation is a fundamental element of empowerment. By participating, people learn skills and experience feelings of self-enhancement that carry over from the specific situation. The experience of success stimulates feelings of self-efficacy and increases the internal locus of control. Participation in collective action can also raise awareness of how political structures operate and affect the individual concerned. From the process point of view, participation has an instrumental function, in that it is a means towards empowerment. From the 'state' point of view, participation is an end towards empowerment, that is, a goal in its own right. It contributes to both psychological and community empowerment. For an in-depth discussion of empowerment processes, we refer to Narayan (2002).

7.5 Approaches in community action

Intersectoral collaboration and community participation are part of what is called 'community action for health'. Nutbeam (1998) defines community action as *collective efforts, which are directed towards increasing community control over the determinants of health, and thereby improving health*. Based on what we have delineated in the previous sections, this definition presumes a situation in which organisations representing a variety of sectors, together with community members, are involved in needs assessment, priority setting, and in the development, implementation and evaluation of actions aiming at the enhancement of health. Theoretically, it assumes shared responsibility, equal power, and an equal voice in decision making. In reality however, within each community visible differences in status and power exist. It also presumes that community action is linked with bottom-up approaches. Yet in practice, we often observe that the work in community-based projects is professional-led, and that levels of participation by citizens are quite low. In this regard it is helpful to consider the different forms that participation can take. Different typologies have been developed to define degrees of community participation, but we will rely on Pretty's (1995) typology of participation, which is based on Arnstein's (1971) eight-rung ladder of participation and presented in Table 7.1. The top of this ladder reflects a purely bottom-up approach. Community members have full control, whereas professionals have only a supporting role. The bottom of the ladder reflects a purely top-down approach, in which professionals have full control: there is no participation. Arnstein (1971) would refer to this situation as manipulation. It should be noted that these levels of participation also apply to intersectoral collaboration. Just consider what happens if we change the word 'people' for organisations or institutions, and 'professionals' for initiating organisations.

It is not so easy to arrive at a bottom-up approach. This is because, on the one hand, community members are quite often not used to participating or working with professionals. On the other hand, most professionals are not used to working with laypeople. Usually,

Table 7.1 Typology of participation (Pretty, 1995).

Levels of participation	
6. Self-mobilisation	Professionals take a back seat in the programme. People make independent decisions, develop their own contacts, and have full control over planning and implementation of activities. Main funding found by people, who have control over its allocation.
5. Interactive participation	People involved in a partnership with professionals in planning and implementing activities. Decisions are made jointly and people contribute resources.
4. Functional participation	People are more involved in the decision- making process. Involved in developing programme and activities. Professionals still have control and make final decisions.
3. Participation by consultation	People are consulted over the programme and their views are listened to and acted upon if thought necessary by the professionals. Decision-making role lies with professionals.
2. Participation by information	People are informed about the programme and activities by asking and answering questions.
1. Passive participation	Professionals have full control over the programme, planning and organising activities, making contacts and taking responsibility for funding. People are informed of plans.
0. No participation	People are not informed about plans; only about activities they are involved in.

professionals are trained in top-down approaches: working on the community instead of working with the community. Additionally, as Laverack and Labonte (2000) argue, this top-down approach is frequently reflected in the professional's job description, as well as in funding mechanisms. This is our experience too. In applying for funding for a community-based health promotion project in one of the Dutch 'big cities', the funding agency obliged the applicants to describe explicitly the health behaviours at which the programme would aim. Consequently, topics had to be decided upon before the involvement in the programme not only of community members, but also of several stake-holding organisations. An interesting concept in relation to this is a 'typology of social change', originating from Rogers and Schoemaker (1971) and adapted by Tones and Tilford (1994). Rogers and Schoemaker distinguished two dimensions in the innovation-change process, one reflecting the origin of the innovation, and the other reflecting the recognition of the need for change. A combination of these dimensions results in four basic change situations. This is presented in Figure 7.1.

a. *Immanent change* happens spontaneously, without any outside intervention. It occurs when the community has a particular felt *and* recognised need for change. In addition, the community itself (or members thereof) invents a solution, and thus the origin of the new idea is internal to the social system. For example, a group of parents may recognise that their children have to cross a dangerous road to

Recognition of need for change \ Origin of new idea	**Internal** to social system	**External** to social system
Internal by members of the social system	(a) Immanent change	(b) Selective contact change
External by change agents outside the social system	(c) Induced immanent change	(d) Direct contact change

Figure 7.1 Types of social change (from Rogers & Schoemaker, 1971).

get to school. They invent and implement the solution of 'cross-over help' where parents take that duty by rotation. In relation to the 'ladder of participation', immanent change is comparable to level 6: self-mobilisation.

b. *Selective contact change* occurs when the community recognises a problem, but an outside source provides a solution. So, if we again take the dangerous road example, the solution is not invented by the parents themselves but by, for example, the municipality or the police. Examples we previously mentioned of issues addressed by community members, such as stress, can also be placed in this category. It compares to interactive (level 5) and functional participation (level 4).

c. *Induced immanent change* occurs when the recognition of the need comes from outside the social system, but where the origin of the new idea comes from inside the system. Outside people help the social system to discover that they have a need and stimulate them to identify what they must do to satisfy that need. This situation occurs, for example, when community developers seek to raise community awareness about unmet needs and then facilitate the acquisition of competencies necessary for the fulfilment of those needs (Tones & Tilford, 1994). Health professionals making a community aware of high levels of cardiovascular disease in a community and trying to involve the community in seeking solutions to address this problem is an example. It reflects participation by consultation (level 3) and participation by information (level 2).

d. *Direct contact change* is the opposite of immanent change (a). In this situation, an external agency decides that the social system has a need or a problem and also provides the solution to that problem or need. Consider a local health organisation that recognises that smoking is a problem in a community (e.g. derived from epidemiological data) and provides the community with 'quit smoking programmes', without actual consultation of their target group. Participation is passive (level 1) or non-existent (level 0).

The condition in quadrant (a) reflects a purely bottom-up approach; the condition in quadrant (d) a typical top-down approach. In terms of 'rate of adoption', it can be expected that the speed of change is fastest in (a), gradually reducing to very slow, or even no adoption at all, in (d). Theoretically, conventional disease prevention programmes have more characteristics of the fourth quadrant, whereas community development programmes adopting the empowerment approach have more characteristics of the selective contact change quadrant. In practice however, health professionals may shift in their approaches and, indeed, combine them.

We can conclude that community-based work is not necessarily synonymous with community participation, or with the 'bottom-up approach'. According to Rifkin *et al.* (2000), it is necessary to make a distinction between mobilisation and involvement. *Mobilisation* means 'getting people to do what professionals think best' and is comparable to induced immanent change (quadrant c). *Involvement* means having people actively decide what they think is best and having professionals contribute expertise and resources to implement this decision and is thus comparable to quadrant (b), selective contact change. Mobilisation thus is more top-down, whereas involvement is more bottom-up.

In Table 7.2 we give an overview of key differences between the top-down and bottom-up approaches, as derived from Laverack and Labonte (2000). It should be noted that the differences are ideal-typical. Several examples are known in which a combination of approaches is followed. External programme initiators initially decide upon the issues to be addressed in community-based programmes, and community participation is of the mobilisation type. This was also our experience in the European food and shopping programme, Super, a nutrition promotion programme conducted in eight European cities, aiming at the reduction of nutrition-related diseases, such as cardiovascular diseases and cancers (Vaandrager *et al.*, 1994; Vaandrager, 1995; Koelen *et al.*, 2001). The project emphasised the importance of intersectoral collaboration and community participation as a strategy for improving public nutrition. In spite of this, professionals initiated the programme. They decided beforehand that the topic was nutrition. The first activities were developed and implemented by a programme team, also consisting of mainly professionals. In the course of the programme, however, increasing numbers of public and voluntary organisations became involved, and people became interested in nutrition. Citizens actively began to request action, initiated new ideas, and started to participate in the development, implementation and evaluation of the programme, thus reaching the level of involvement.

Table 7.2 *Key differences between top-down and bottom-up approaches.*

	Top-down	Bottom-up
Root/metaphor	Individual responsibility	Empowerment
Approach/orientation	Weakness/deficit	Strength/capacity
	Solve problems	Improve competence
Definition of problem	By outside agent such as government body	By community
Primary vehicles for health promotion and change	Education, improved services. Lifestyle	Building community control, resources and capacities towards economic, social and political change
Role of outside agents	Service delivery and resource allocation	Respond to needs of community
Primary decision makers	Agency representatives, business leaders, 'appointed community leaders'	Indigenous appointed leaders
Community control of resources	Low	High
Community ownership	Low	High
Evaluation	Specific risk factors	Pluralistic methods documenting changes of importance to the community

Based on Laverack & Labonte, 2000

Similar experiences are reported for community-based health promotion programmes such as the North Karelia project on cardiovascular disease (Puska *et al.*, 1985), and in Heart Beat Wales (Nutbeam & Catfort, 1987). In our opinion, participation has to be considered as a dynamic process moving along the continuum from no participation to self-mobilisation, but not necessarily forwards.

7.6 The 'how' of community action

The cornerstone of intersectoral collaboration and community is joint working, that is, the process of working together to achieve a common goal, irrespective of the boundaries of the different organisations and sectors. The added value of collective action is generally acknowledged. Positive claims in favour of this approach include that it:

- focuses on the promotion of health of populations instead of on individuals or groups at risk;
- reflects the awareness that infrastructure and social norms influence individual behaviour;
- encourages organisations, decision makers and politicians to consider the health consequences of their policies;
- increases sense of ownership of programmes by communities;
- leads to empowerment at individual and community level; and
- makes a firm contribution to decreasing socio-economic differences in health.

Community action for health can take many different forms. As we mentioned in the previous section, it usually begins with a core group of concerned professionals and/or concerned citizens that initiate an action process. One of the most mentioned formats is that of community coalitions. From the several definitions that aim to describe community coalitions, we can derive the following essential characteristics. They can be either formal or informal alliances of individuals, representing diverse organisations, diverse interest groups, diverse actions or diverse constituencies, which combine their human and material resources and are directed at achieving common goals that the members are unable to achieve independently.

We are able to describe three types of coalitions, based on membership: grassroots coalitions, professional coalitions and coalitions of professional and grassroots leaders (*cf.* Feighery & Rogers, 1989). *Grassroots coalitions* are organised by volunteers in times of crisis to pressure policy makers to act. They have the characteristics of pressure groups, which are voluntary groups of individuals linked by shared goals, and who attempt to obtain decisions and actions favourable to their goals. They can use various means, but in particular proceed by exerting influence on governments or other decision-making units (*cf.* Bracht & Tsouris, 1990). Examples of grassroots coalitions are a group of community members who want to oppose the closing of a community centre in a neighbourhood, a group of parents advocating a safe cycle path from their residential area to school, or a group of workers pressing for a smoke-free work environment. *Professional coalitions* are formed by professional organisations, either in times of crisis or as a long-term approach to increasing their power and influence. An example of this type of coalition is Tobacco Free America, organised by the American Cancer Society and the American Lung Association to influence tobacco issues (Butterfoss *et al.*, 1993). *Coalitions of professionals and grassroots leaders* in communities are formed to influence more long-term health and welfare practices for their communities. Such coalitions are usually initiated by one or more agencies in response to funding proposals. In fact, this type of coalition is comparable to what Bracht and Gleason (1990) call the 'leadership board or council model', in which existing leaders and/or community activists work together towards a common goal, such as smoke-free environments or accident prevention. The types of coalitions are not static. It is possible for grassroots coalitions to become mixed coalitions. A good example of this is the Foundation Against 'Senseless Violence' in The Netherlands. The foundation was established in 1997 and represents action groups initiated by groups of people who have lost a relative (child, sibling, friend, neighbour) in an act of violence. Today, the Foundation works together with several professional organisations such as the police, youth organisations, popular radio stations, and nightclub organisations in the struggle against social violence (*Landelijke Stichting Tegen Zinloos Geweld*, 2002). Usually however, health promotion programmes begin as professional coalitions, and then become mixed coalitions, especially those programmes that can be placed in quadrant (c) of Figure 7.1, in which problems are identified by 'experts' and where those professionals recruit members of the community to assist in solving these problems. The previously mentioned Super project is an example of this. Similar examples are the Pawtucket Heart Health Programme (Roncarati *et al.*, 1989), the Minnesota Heart Health Programme (Luepker *et al.*, 1994), and the North Karelia Project (Puska *et al.*, 1985). From literature it is clear that coalitions become increasingly formal in structure as the number of professionals involved increases. Therefore it is probably better to talk about consortia, which tend to be relatively professional in nature and are mostly linked to organisations in a formal way.

7.7 Barriers to collective community action

In almost all literature about community action it is mentioned that it is difficult to arrive at a good balance between both community participation and intersectoral collaboration. This seems to be particularly true in programmes that are characterised by induced immanent change. The literature often deals with either community participation or intersectoral collaboration. In our opinion however, the concepts are very much the same. Central to both is participation in joint programmes, regardless of whether the participants represent formal organisations or community groups. Consequently, any barriers experienced are often applicable to both. Yet, there are some differences. For this reason we firstly address barriers that are reported in the literature relating to community participation, and then the barriers reported in intersectoral collaboration.

7.7.1 Barriers to community participation

To arrive at a fair level of community participation in health promotion is a noble aspiration, but it also appears to be a difficult one. Clearly, simply approaching community members and asking them to participate in project planning and implementation proves unsuccessful (Koelen, 2000). In several publications addressing this issue, reference is made to low levels of public participation, to lack of public access to decision making, or to professional dominance. Even though many projects start from the idea of active community participation, quite often these projects lead to frustration because professionals frequently seem unable to put these principles into practice. Armed with, for example, epidemiological data, professionals point out that at least changes in behaviours conducive to health have to be achieved (e.g. nutrition, smoking, exercise, alcohol) and therefore implicitly work according to a top-down approach. Experience from several community-based health promotion programmes (*cf.* Koelen *et al.*, 2001; Wagemakers & Koelen, 2001; Maeland & Haglund, 1999; Wallerstein, 1999; Sullivan *et al.*, 2001; De Haes *et al.*, 2002; Voorham *et al.*, 2002) shows that people express needs far beyond those behaviours. People often prefer to work on issues relating to stress, feelings of security, housing conditions, or social interactions, or else to engage in practical projects such as building play facilities for children and restoring community centres. Health professionals often disregard these needs. It should be realised that people generally consider their lives from a holistic perspective, whereas professionals tend to focus on specific (health-impairing) issues. This tendency is probably due to the fact that professionals are trained in a reductionist tradition, that is, in specific fields, and in specialised subjects. Moreover, professionals are held accountable for what they do. In order to get the 'go ahead' for a project, the organisations they represent (or indeed funding agencies) have to be convinced of the necessity of the project and of the health benefits to be gained. A precondition then is that the interventions aim at indicators against which performance can be measured, such as increased knowledge, positive changes in attitudes or self-efficacy, in relation to a specific behaviour. So, it is understandable that professionals take a specialist stance, but we should regard this with caution. A reductionist approach increases the chance of the focus being on symptoms of ill health, instead of on their causes. Theoretically, health promotion adopts a holistic approach to health. In Chapter 2 we related this conception of health to Maslow's hierarchy of needs, in which it is stated that more complex needs become important only after the more basic needs have been satisfied. Amongst these basic needs are physiological needs (hunger, thirst) and safety needs (including housing and a safe environment). Therefore, a broad engagement is clearly in line with the philosophy underlying health promotion. In fact, broad issues such as feelings of security, housing conditions, and stress can be used as an entry point to get specific topics onto the agenda. For example, it is generally known that psychological stress is related to behaviours like smoking, alcohol, and physical exercise.

Several additional barriers to participation are identified in the literature (see for example Cook *et al.*, 1988; Wandersman & Giamartino, 1980; Bracht & Tsourus, 1990; Altman *et al.*, 1991). A first group of factors is related to what we might call a *lack of knowledge*. This includes a lack of individual and community awareness of the existence of a health problem, a lack of problem-solving capacities, and ignorance about how to gain access to information. A second group of factors relates to a *lack of social cohesion*. In fact, this refers to those aspects that bind groups or societies together, such as feelings of belonging to a community, and feelings of inter-relatedness (see section 4.2.2). The weaker these factors, the more difficult it is to establish community participation. Wandersman and Giamartino (1980), for example, found that participation of community members was more likely to occur among those who where concerned about their neighbourhood, had more experience in community leadership, and felt that competent colleagues could be enlisted to support the project. Ecklund (1999), in her evaluation of two community-based health promotion projects in Finland, also found that 'sense of community' was an important factor in enabling community participation, as was interest and commitment from power holders and decision makers. A possible cause for low levels of social cohesion can probably be found in what we said before about the tendency of professionals to define the community from the outsider's perspective. This underlines the importance of finding out whether the people aimed at indeed consider themselves to be a community. A third problem is that of misunderstanding and *conflicts that arise between laypeople and experts*. On the one hand, this is related to the type of knowledge on which problem definitions and decisions are based: scientifically validated knowledge, most often used by the professionals, and knowledge by experience, most often used by laypeople. Scientific knowledge is usually considered to be more valuable than knowledge by experience (Koelen, 1992). In addition, professionals frequently seem to have difficulty accepting the views and knowledge of community representatives. Illustrative of this point are phrases found in the literature, in which the importance is emphasised of 'ensuring that participating citizens are well trained', or 'training community representatives so that they may better understand how experts approach problems'. No reference is then made to the necessity of changing the professionals' attitudes, or of training the professionals in the acquisition of new skills needed to handle the new roles they have to play. Furthermore, in situations where both the problem and the solution have been identified by external experts (see Figure 7.1, quadrant d), it often seems to be difficult to convince community members and to motivate them to take part in action (*cf.* Clark *et al.*, 1993)

7.7.2 Barriers to intersectoral collaboration

Organisations are generally designed for specifically described aims and objectives. They develop their own philosophy, their own culture, their own value and norm system, and their own rituals. For a long time the main tendency was to establish highly specialised organisations, with a clear focus. It is no different for health organisations. We have organisations focusing on specific parts of the body, such as the heart or kidneys. Other organisations focus on specific issues, such as nutrition or alcohol. Others again serve specific age groups, such as organisations for the elderly. We can expect that collaboration with other organisations will be accompanied by difficulties. Clark *et al.* (1993) analysed seven case studies on collaborative efforts to improve the social, economic or health status of residents in poor communities. They identify *problems in collaboration itself*, including fear and distrust of outside organisations, and lack of experience in participatory processes. Besides these, they identify *programme-management problems*, including lack of leadership, ineffective formal procedures or policies, and weak structures for inter-organisational communication. Another difficulty that is often mentioned relates to a lack of official or political support. This includes a lack of faith on the part of sponsoring groups or agencies, difficulties in obtaining finance for the work, lack of official and political commitment, and lack of 'social' support.

Barriers are also reported in relation to the way programmes are developed and implemented (*cf.* Kreuter *et al.*, 2000; Graham & Bois, 1997; Koelen, 2000; Wagemakers & Koelen, 2001; Voorham *et al.*, 2002; Goosen *et al.*, 2004). Firstly, it is difficult to get started and to find a clear definition of roles and responsibilities for each of the participants (organisations or their representatives) in the programme. In practice, programmes are often initiated by a small professional coalition trying to find external funding. Once funding has been obtained, the project has to begin, and the small coalition seeks to expand with related groups and organisations. However, the overall aims and objectives are already spelled out in the funding proposal, and there is often little scope for new participants to have an influence on the direction of the programme. Several (review) studies show that further discussions about the meaning of the predefined aims and objectives almost never take place, due to which expectations about the project and about each other's roles and responsibilities remain unspoken. This strongly hampers the collaboration process, and thereby the project as a whole (*cf.* Goodman *et al.*, 1995; Graham & Bois, 1997; Kreuter *et al.*, 2000; Wagemakers & Koelen, 2001; Goossen *et al.*, 2004). Studies of, for example, Wallerstein (2000), Mendes and Akerman (2001) and Wagemakers (2000) show that, particularly in the start-up phase of health promotion projects, serious conflicts may arise between the collaborating parties. Hence, it is especially important to start projects with open communication and explicit discussion about the 'mission' of the project. The previously mentioned study of Wallerstein (2000) and also Dutch experiences (Wagemakers & Koelen, 2001; Weijters & Koelen, 2002) show that discussions about such conflicts can clear the air, and that the collaboration processes then run smoothly.

Secondly, expectations about outcomes in terms of changes in behaviour and lifestyle, and changes in conditions that affect health status, often appear to be unrealistic. It should be realised that changes do not happen overnight and can often only be reached in the long term. Unrealistic outcome expectations will discourage the sustainability of efforts, since the visibility of results is one of the major stimulating and driving forces to staying on track.

7.8 Challenges in community action

The literature often paints a depressing picture of participatory community action, but the added value is also clear. It is therefore worthwhile giving this subject considerable attention. Despite the difficulties in building networks for collaboration and participation in community-based health promotion, and despite all the conditions necessary to make it into a successful enterprise, the added value it has over single actions of single institutions makes it a challenge into which it is worthwhile investing effort, time and energy. In an evaluation of a community-based project in The Netherlands (Tuveri & Koelen, 1998), participants were asked to list the difficulties and challenges of their intersectoral efforts. Together with the points mentioned above, respondents mentioned that it takes more time than working alone, and that it is difficult to deal with the many different ideas, interests, and ways of working, as well as the different expectations of the parties involved. These difficulties were outweighed however, by positive experiences. According to those interviewed, intersectoral efforts lead to better results, better contacts with other organisations and people, and a broader perspective on the issue concerned. In addition, they mentioned that 'learning from each other', and 'the enthusiasm of the partners in action' strongly stimulates and provides motivation for continued participation in collaboration. The principle of synergy seems to be very strong.

Zakus and Lysack (1998) list predisposing conditions favourable to participation in community action (see Table 7.3). These conditions relate to the political context in which it takes place, the health care delivery system, the experience and skills of the partners involved in working together, and willingness to accept responsibility.

We argue that it is important to scrutinise critically both the opportunities and the constraints of collective action. First of all, we have to mention that it is not the solution to all problems; but secondly, and probably more importantly, we should be aware that it is not a self-generating autonomous phenomenon. On the contrary, it involves a learning process. The way it may spread through a community reflects the way innovations are diffused as we described in Chapter 4. Interdisciplinary projects include a variety of domains. Each domain brings in its own specific knowledge and information content, its own general aims, and its own horizons. Usually they do not have a history of working together on a common goal. All actors have to learn to listen to each other, having respect and consideration for each other's opinions and possibilities. Collective community action thus can be considered from the perspective of adoption of innovations, since it means new ways of working for those involved. As mentioned before, it usually begins with a core group of concerned people that initiate an action process: the innovators. They are not always respected or trusted by others, but they can launch the new idea. When results become visible, early adopters will follow, and gradually the 'change' spreads throughout the community. It should be noted that networks for community action need regular attention (maintenance), because without such attention they are likely to deteriorate. Compare it to a car: to keep it going it needs regular maintenance. Therefore, a clear communication and information structure, good management, and visibility deserve continuous attention. We will elaborate on this topic further in Chapter 10.

Table 7.3 Predisposing conditions for community action in health.

- A political climate that accepts and supports active community participation and interaction at all levels of programme development, implementation and evaluation.
- A political context in which policy, legislation, and resource allocation takes account of regional/local circumstances, aspirations and needs.
- A socio-cultural and political context, which supports individual and collective public awareness, knowledge acquisition and discussion of issues and problems affecting individual and collective wellbeing.
- A political and administrative system, which promotes and accepts decentralisation and regional/local authority for decision making on health policy, resource allocation and programmes.
- An acceptable and universal level of availability and accessibility of health services for meeting basic health care needs on a systematic basis.
- A health care delivery system in which institutions and professionals experience with and are committed to a community orientation through such mechanisms as institutional boards, advisory groups, health committees, and community education programmes.
- A health care delivery system in which the institutions, service professionals and managers are flexible, genuinely committed and supportive, and have experience with attempting to respond to regional/local needs in collaborative and creative ways among themselves and with government.
- Some experience in intersectoral activity of health services and professionals with related services such as water and sanitation, other public works, occupational health, agriculture, social services, housing, and the law.
- A citizenry in possession of sufficient awareness of, and knowledge and skills in social organisation and health related issues.
- A community in which health is a priority issue and which demonstrates widespread interest in healthy lifestyles, fitness, nutrition, disease eradication and prevention, and a safe and healthy environment.
- A community that is willing to collectively accept responsibility, and give their consent and commitment to community health initiatives.
- A community with previous successful experience with community participation.
- Responsible, responsive, and efficient media, information and communication system within and between communities and with various government levels.
- For all concerned, the proposed participation must be perceived as meaningful and leading to prompt, visible results in addition to achievement of important longer term goals.

Source: Zakus & Lysack, 1998: 5.

7.9 Chapter summary

In this chapter we elaborated on the concepts of intersectoral collaboration, community participation, and empowerment, which are considered key strategies in the promotion of health. We then presented different approaches in community action, with in the extremes the top-down (expert-led) and the bottom-up approach (community-led). An interesting concept in relation to this is a typology of social change, in which two dimensions in the change process are distinguished: the origin of the innovation and the recognition of a need for change. Special attention has been paid to barriers in collective community action, and to factors influencing the success and sustainability of such actions. We concluded that achieving and sustaining intersectoral collaboration and community participation is not easy but is certainly worthwhile, since it can create synergy between participating organisations.

8. Designing health education and health promotion

Effective health education and health promotion require systematic planning. This chapter deals with this issue. A planned programme is necessary for single activities, such as the provision of information about a new health service in a factory to a meeting of employees, as well as for activities that might occupy a group of people and organisations for several years, such as a community-based programme to prevent cardiovascular disease. Whatever the situation, decisions need to be made about objectives, people to involve, people to address, strategies for action, the organisation of activities - including the means of financing these activities - and the evaluation plan.

In the course of time, several planning models have been developed. Some of these models are based in the tradition of disease prevention and lifestyle change. The central point is the analysis of health-related behaviour. Other models are formulated in terms of problem analysis in a broader sense, including community diagnosis and organisational setting. Yet other models include aspects of both. Well-known are the Precede-Proceed model (Green & Kreuter, 1991), the five-stage community organisation model for health promotion (Bracht et al., 1999), and intervention mapping (Bartholomew et al., 2001). Although planning models differ in terminology, they generally consist of four logical phases: diagnosis, programme development, implementation, and evaluation (see Figure 8.1).

In the diagnosis phase, problems and needs are identified and analysed. In the programme development phase, concrete activities are

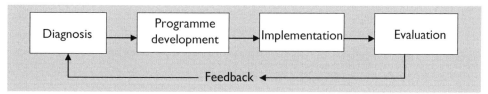

Figure 8.1 Phases in planning and evaluation.

developed. In the implementation phase, the planned activities are put into practice. Evaluation is concerned with finding out whether the implemented activities have been successful. In this chapter, we will address each planning phase by formulating the important questions to be answered and the decisions to be made. We should realise that planning is not a strict sequential procedure. For example, evaluation is positioned at the end, whereas in fact evaluation has to be considered from the very onset of planning. The whole can best be conceived as an iterative process: in each phase we both look back to the previous phases and look forward to the following phases. We will describe each phase separately for the sake of clarity.

Throughout the phases in planning, theories that have been presented in previous chapters can help to clarify or describe problems and to identify possibilities for addressing these problems. Research also plays an important role in guiding and evaluating this process. In this chapter we refer to research only superficially; this subject will be addressed in the following chapter in more detail. We are aware that to separate research from planning is somehow artificial, since in practice action and research are often interwoven. Research aims not only to analyse a situation and its problems, but also to find solutions to these problems. This requires a research approach in which results are immediately fed back into the project. In the previous chapter, we argued that health education or health promotion programmes might be initiated by different persons, groups or organisations. If the need for action emerges directly from the community, participants will feel more involved and will be more prone to participate actively than when the need for action is identified by some professional or external agency. It is recommended, though, that members of the community or target population become involved as early as possible in each stage and, whenever possible, also in the research.

Before we proceed with planning, we will firstly elaborate on objectives. Objectives are essential in each phase. They are formulated in the diagnosis and programme development phase, and evaluated in the implementation and evaluation phase. Statements about the effectiveness and efficiency of any programme are always related to the question of whether the objectives have been met.

8.1 Objectives

In health education and health promotion, as in any other professional field, we frequently talk about 'what we want to achieve'. A variety of terms are used to describe the results of programmes. Reference is made to missions, purposes, aims, objectives, goals, and targets. However, there is no universal agreement about the meaning of the various statements. We propose to use a *hierarchy of objectives* defined as follows:

- *Health objectives* describe health issues to be addressed, for whom (target group), which health benefit should be achieved, and within what timeframe.
- *Behavioural objectives* contain specific behaviour to be addressed. This can be either one type of behaviour or a number of behaviours. For example, cardiovascular disease is influenced by behaviours such as smoking, nutrition, and physical exercise.
- *Environmental objectives* spell out those conditions in the environment necessary to facilitate or support behavioural change. They include such aspects as economic factors, policy, legislation, and the organisation of health services.
- *Intervention objectives* define cognitive (e.g. knowledge, beliefs, attitudes) and psychomotor (skills) elements that will be addressed in the intervention. In addition, they specify the environmental conditions that should be achieved or attained in order to facilitate and enable the planned change.
- *Programme objectives* describe the specific activities that will be conducted in order to achieve the intervention objectives. They refer to message content, communication methods, strategies and channels to be used, and the settings in which the action takes place.
- *Process objectives* refer to the organisation of the programme and resources necessary to implement the programme. They are formulated in terms such as collaboration structures, material, manpower, time and financial resources.

These six categories of objectives differ in terms of specificity, and in the time needed to achieve them. The objectives at the top of the hierarchy are formulated in overall achievement terms and are often based on long-term expectations. These objectives are elaborated down the hierarchy into a widening set of more specific objectives, more operational, more short-run, and more measurable. The objectives further down the hierarchy offer the operational criteria for evaluation. However, it often appears to be difficult to formulate objectives in a clear way. Five criteria have been suggested for the design and specification of high quality objectives: the so-called SMART criteria (Simnett, 1995). Objectives should be:

S Specific (to a disease, a social group, age, or geographical location);
M Measurable (using important indicators);
A Agreed upon by all concerned;
R Realistic (achievable within resource and other constraints);
T Time bound (achievable within a timescale).

Objectives also have to express realistic expectations of the change that is expected. Based on the notions of stages of change and on the diffusion of innovations theory (see Chapter 4), it is not realistic to expect 100 per cent change in any population. But what is success? Green and Lewis (1986) identify four kinds of standards that might be used to determine the relative success of a given intervention.

1. *Historical standards*: expectations can be derived from successes of previous and comparable programmes. For example, for a stop-smoking programme that has previously been applied in other settings with a success rate of 15 per cent after 6 months, it is realistic to expect a 15 per cent success rate in the new programme too.

2. *Normative standards*: expectations based on the level of performance achieved by other workers in programmes of a similar nature and designed for similar target groups.

3. *Theoretical standards*: expectations derived from knowledge of relevant theory. This refers to what one might reasonably expect in the light of a conceptual analysis based on previous research in a given area, as well as to interventions that have been piloted under controlled experimental conditions.

4. *Absolute standards*: expectation of 100 per cent success.

The formulation of objectives needs serious consideration throughout the diagnosis and programme development phases. Objectives give direction to the programme and its specific activities. Moreover, they offer the criteria against which the activities and programmes are evaluated in the implementation and evaluation phase. How they relate to each phase will be discussed in the remainder of this chapter.

8.2 Diagnosis

Planning begins with a systematic assessment of health problems and of the possibilities for addressing these problems. We will deal with this phase extensively, because sophisticated diagnosis is half the battle. In practice, we often find that professionals are prone to look at a problem quickly and then select a strategy in order to address that problem. The *how question* then dominates the *why question*. In order to reduce or solve a problem however, we need to know *why* the problem exists, and we need to know the *causes* of this problem. Otherwise we end up with actions that focus on symptoms instead of on their causes. Taking the why question as the point of departure increases the chances of the resulting programme suiting the problem and the possibilities, and therefore increases effectiveness.

Diagnosis consists of three domains of activity: diagnosis of the situation in which the problem occurs, diagnosis of its behavioural and environmental causes, and diagnosis of the determinants of these causes. Each domain diagnosis results in the formulation of objectives. We will highlight the important questions to be answered and the information needed to answer these questions. We illustrate the steps with two examples: cardiovascular disease and road traffic accidents.

8.2.1 Diagnosis of the existing situation

The diagnosis phase begins with a description of the health situation of a given population, for example a group of patients, students, adolescents, young mothers, schools, or a residential area in a city. Information is required about aspects that positively and negatively influence the quality of life of the population under study. It includes their perceived needs, subjectively defined problems, perceived priorities and challenges. In addition, epidemiological data about the health status of the population, and social indicators such as unemployment, education levels, crime rates, overcrowding, and mental health are relevant. This information gives some idea of the quality of life in the population, the existence and extent of possible health problems, and specific groups or individuals within that population who are probably most affected. It should be noted that, in many situations, persons other than those involved in developing programmes to address problems initially identify these problems. For example, an epidemiologist may find that in certain areas the incidence of cancers is higher than in others, paediatricians may observe an increase in obese children, school management may observe an increasing number of students that gamble, community nurses may observe that elderly people do not feel safe enough to go for a walk in their own neighbourhood. This means that health promotion workers become involved after problems have been described and defined. If this is the case, we recommend careful examination of the information on which the problem definition is based.

In community-based programmes it is important to involve community members and representatives of major sectors in the community, such as health, education, recreation, business, religious, statutory and voluntary organisations, in the diagnosis phase. They possess important information about the community's social structure, and about the community's health and behaviour patterns. What is more, early involvement creates more possibilities for gaining support for the programme.

Diagnosis of the existing situation provides information on which priorities can be set for educational and promotional efforts. These priorities are described in health objectives. *Health objectives* describe the health issues to be addressed, for whom (target group), which health benefit should be achieved, within what timeframe. Examples are:
- A reduction of 10 per cent in the prevalence of cardiovascular disease in the male population, in the 40 to 60 age group, in a certain community within the next five years, or,
- A reduction of 25 per cent in the number of children hospitalised due to road traffic accidents in a specified geographic area within the next three years.

In line with the principle of active community participation, community members should play a visible role in setting priorities. As stated in section 7.7.1, we should be conscious that discrepancies often appear between the perception of community members and the perception of health professionals regarding the most urgent problems to address. We cannot offer a blueprint for handling such a situation, but wish to emphasise that ignoring the priorities as set by community members will seriously hamper the participation process and reduce the effectiveness of the programme.

Diagnosis of the existing situation provides the general framework for action. The steps are summarised in Table 8.1.

Table 8.1 Summary of phases, activities, and objectives.

Phase	Activities	Objectives
Diagnosis of existing situation	• assessment of perceived needs and priorities	→ Health objectives
	• examination of epidemiological data and social indicators	
	• setting priorities for action	
→ objectives to be formulated		

8.2.2 Diagnosis of behavioural and environmental causes

We precede the diagnosis with an assessment of the behavioural and environmental factors that are related to the defined health problem.

Behavioural diagnosis is a systematic analysis of the behavioural links to the health problem. Health issues are often related to groups of behaviours. For example, cardiovascular diseases are related to behaviours such as smoking, alcohol consumption, nutrition, physical exercise, and stress. Generally it is impossible to address all these behaviours in one programme due to time constraints, so a selection needs to be made. We propose, as do Green and Kreuter (1991), rating the behaviours in terms of importance and estimated changeability. The *importance of a behaviour* in relation to a health issue can be derived from existing scientific knowledge. Ratings of *changeability* of behaviour can often be based on results that have been achieved by other programmes and previous research. It should be realised that some behaviours are less susceptible to change than others. For example, behaviours that are rooted in culture, behaviours with a high level of repetition (as is the case with habits), and addictive behaviours are often difficult to change. This is not to say that these behaviours are not changeable, but it will take considerable time and special conditions. Importance and changeability rates produce a matrix of behaviours, as illustrated in Figure 8.2. Behavioural diagnosis provides the information necessary in order to formulate *behavioural objectives*.

Examples of behavioural objectives are:
- A reduction of 15 per cent in the number of smokers in the defined male population within the next two years.
- A 30 per cent increase in physical exercise up to a level of 15 minutes of physical activity a day in the defined population within two years.
- A decrease in fat intake to a level of 30 per cent of total daily calorie intake within one year.

Note that behavioural objectives can also apply to persons other than the actual target group. For instance, in reducing children's road traffic accidents, the behaviour of parents as well as of car drivers is important. Behavioural objectives can then be:
- Within one year, 40 per cent of parents will have bought cycle helmets for their children.
- Within one year, 20 per cent of children will wear helmets when cycling in traffic.
- Within one year, 50 per cent of the car drivers in the specific area will have reduced their speed from 50 to 30 km an hour.

Environmental diagnosis focuses on aspects in the physical and social environment that are linked to health issues (Green & Kreuter, 1991). We use the term 'environment' to refer to those external aspects that (1) directly influence a person's health, such as noise, air and water pollution; (2) enable or constrain health behaviour, such as the

	More important	Less important
More changeable	High priority for programme focus (1)	(3)
Less changeable	(2)	No programme (4)

Figure 8.2 Matrix of health behaviours (Green & Kreuter, 1991).

availability and accessibility of services (including access to information), and possibilities for recreation; and (3) involve the political and organisational situation, such as health policy, and health protective legislation and regulation. As with behaviour, environmental aspects can be rated in terms of importance and changeability. Environmental diagnosis results in the formulation of *environmental objectives*, which spell out the conditions in the environment that need to be changed. For example:

- A change in policy, e.g. introducing a no-smoking policy in a workplace.
- The provision of sports facilities in a factory.

Or, in the second example,

- The provision of safe areas for children to play in.
- Legislation aimed at reducing maximum speed in an area.

We expand Table 8.1 with behavioural and environmental diagnosis and continue with the last step in the diagnosis phase.

Table 8.2 Summery of phases, activities, and objectives.

Phase	Activities	Objectives
Diagnosis of existing situation	• assessment of perceived needs and priorities • examination of epidemiological data and social indicators • setting priorities for action	→ Health objectives
Diagnosis of behavioural causes	• analysis of behavioural links with health problem • ratings of importance and changeability	→ Behavioural objectives
Diagnosis of environmental causes	• analysis of environmental links with the health problem • ratings of importance and changeability	→ Environmental objectives
→ objectives to be formulated		

8.2.3 Diagnosis of determinants of behavioural and environmental causes

So far, several decisions have been made in the diagnosis phase. One is inclined to think that it is now 'time to take action'. However, this decision has to be postponed. There is one more pivotal step to go in diagnosis. As we mentioned in Chapter 3, it is one thing to know that a particular behaviour negatively affects health, but quite another thing to know how to change such behaviour. The same is true for environmental conditions. Insight into *why people behave as they do*, and into *why the environmental conditions are as they are*, is needed in order to know *how* to change behaviour, and *how* to influence the environmental conditions. Hence, we need to analyse the selected behavioural and environmental conditions further in terms of their determinants.

Diagnosis of behavioural determinants
Individual behaviour cannot always be explained straightforwardly. All too often it is assumed that a lack of knowledge is the major cause for people continuing with health-impairing behaviour. In Chapters 3 and 4, we described how behaviour depends on such determinants as knowledge, awareness, attitudes, social influence, perceived control, and environmental conditions. Moreover, someone can be aware of the health risk of a certain behaviour but have not yet decided to change. Or a person may have made a number of attempts but consistently failed to succeed, and this consistent failure may have led to stable internal attributions (lack of ability). Different determinants require different action. A comprehensive examination of determinants of behaviour is necessary to provide clear indicators in order to induce change. Green and Kreuter (1991) divide the determinants of behaviour into three groups:
- *Predisposing factors* relate to the motivation of an individual or group to act. These determinants are psychological or cognitive in nature, and include such variables as awareness, knowledge, beliefs and attitudes, perceived needs, and perceived abilities (i.e. self-efficacy).
- *Reinforcing factors* are those that determine whether the individual or group receives positive or negative feedback and support. Positive incentives contribute to persistence or repetition. Incentives may be social in nature, for example a supportive social environment, including family, peers, employers, health care

providers, community leaders and decision makers. They may also be physical in nature, for example experiencing weight loss while dieting, an increased feeling of wellbeing after physical exercise, or pain relief after following a recommended therapy.

- *Enabling factors* facilitate the motivation to take action. They include aspects relating to the individual, such as the skills that are needed to carry out behavioural change. They also include environmental conditions, such as the availability and affordability of resources, and the accessibility of services.

Diagnosis of environmental determinants

Environmental aspects are part of the enabling factors but deserve attention in their own right, since they can either hinder or stimulate behaviour change. For example, we can determine whether local shops include low fat products in their range of goods offered, the pricing of such products, the availability and accessibility of sports facilities, opening hours of these facilities, and cost of membership. Information about existing policies, and the possibilities for changing such policies, is also important. Policy change is often beyond the control of health professionals, but they can strongly advocate stimulating policy change. For example, they can address the issue of a dangerous road crossing in a residential area to a councillor of the municipality.

Setting priorities

In order to set priorities, behavioural and environmental determinants can again be rated in terms of importance and changeability (see Figure 8.2). Firstly, priority has to be established among the groups of predisposing, reinforcing and enabling factors. For example, if people are unaware of the health risks of certain behaviours, it is not helpful to focus on skills. Likewise, to promote condom use is worthless, and even unethical, if condoms are not available or not affordable. Secondly, priority has to be established within the groups.

The *intervention objectives* can then be formulated based on the priorities. Intervention objectives define the cognitive (learning) and psychomotor (skills) elements that will be addressed in the intervention, and they specify the environmental conditions that should be achieved or attained in order to facilitate and enable the planned change. For example, within one year:

- 70 Per cent of the defined male population will be aware that physical exercise is an important contributory factor to the reduction of cardiovascular disease.
- 50 Per cent will have a positive attitude towards practising physical exercise.
- 30 Per cent will have the skills to increase physical exercise.
- The majority of employers will provide either sports facilities at work, or possibilities for employees to use the facilities of a nearby sports centre during working hours.

Or, in relation to the objective 'within one year, car drivers in a specific area will have reduced their speed from 50 to 30 km an hour':
- All car drivers in the specified area will be aware of the dangers involved in fast driving in the neighbourhood.
- 80 Per cent of car drivers will be motivated to reduce their speed.
- Environmental measures will be taken to discourage car drivers from speeding.

Note that intervention objectives express concisely what is to be achieved and are formulated in specific terms. This is necessary because they provide the criteria against which the outcomes of a programme are evaluated. As can be seen in the example, the percentages of expected change decrease in the subsequent statements. Often a relatively high proportion of a given population can be made aware of a fact, but a smaller proportion will believe that the fact is relevant or important to them, and a still smaller proportion will develop the necessary skills to carry out the recommended actions, and a smaller proportion again will actually carry out the recommended action. The activities in the diagnosis of behavioural and environmental determinants are summarised in Table 8.3.

8.3 Programme development

The programme development phase is basically directed at the translation of the intervention objectives into action. It includes (1) building networks for collective action; (2) selection of the best ways of achieving the objectives at environmental and individual level; more specifically, the selection of strategies, messages, channels, and settings; (3) the organisation of activities, including identification of

Table 8.3 Summery of phases, activities, and objectives.

Phase	Activities	Objectives
Diagnosis of existing situation	• assessment of perceived needs and priorities • examination of epidemiological data and social indicators • setting priorities for action	→ Health objectives
Diagnosis of behavioural causes	• analysis of behavioural links with health problem • ratings of importance and changeability	→ Behavioural objectives
Diagnosis of environmental causes	• analysis of environmental links with the health problem • ratings of importance and changeability	→ Environmental objectives

Diagnosis of behavioural and environmental determinants	• analysis of determinants of behaviour in terms of its predisposing, reinforcing and enabling factors
	• analysis of environmental determinants
	• setting priorities
		→ Intervention objectives
		  • cognitive and psychomotoric
		  • environmental conditions

→ objectives to be formulated

necessary resources; and (4) setting a clear programme plan. The programme development phase consists of two types of objectives, programme objectives and process objectives.

8.3.1 Building networks for collective action

In health promotion projects, activities involving community members and relevant organisations need considerable attention (see Chapter 7). This includes identifying and contacting individuals who may wish to participate in the programme. Key informants, who have been involved in diagnosis, can be recruited for programme development and implementation. Generally, these representatives should be people who can speak and make decisions for the organisations or people they represent (Bracht *et al.*, 1999). Working relationships need to be established, and it is important to clarify roles and responsibilities, taking into account individual abilities, expectations, and interests. It could be a condition that participants in the programme acquire competence in a certain subject. Consider the role of laypeople, paraprofessionals and peer educators. But learning new competencies also applies to professionals. In section 7.7.1 we argued that it might be necessary to train professionals in the new roles they have to play. With appropriate information and guidance, community members and professionals create partnerships and are able to plan and conduct effective programmes for their community.

8.3.2 Selection of intervention strategies

Developing a programme implies that decisions have to be made about strategies through which change can be achieved. Consideration needs to be given as to how the issues to be addressed fit within national or local policies, how they fit within community organisations, how they relate to existing activities, etc. For a detailed description of assessment of community organisations, policies, and regulations, refer to Bracht *et al.* (1999) and Green and Kreuter (1991). We wish to address two specific issues here. Firstly, we look at instruments that may be selected for inducing change. Subsequently, we describe some criteria for the development of communicative interventions.

Intervention mix
Intervention objectives define cognitive and psychomotor elements that will be addressed in the intervention. In addition, they specify the environmental conditions that should be achieved or attained in order to facilitate and enable planned change. Communicative interventions alone will generally not be sufficient to achieve these objectives. Considering the complexity of behaviour and the environment in which the behaviour takes place, a combination of instruments is usually required. This is illustrated in Figure 8.3.

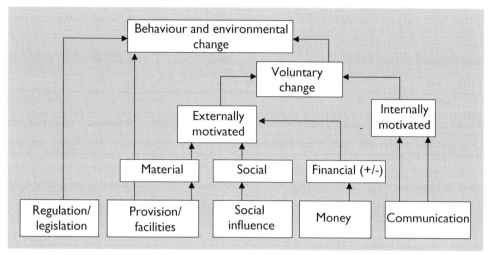

Figure 8.3   Behavioural and environmental change instruments (based on van Woerkum et al., 1999).

Consider the intervention objectives relating to the reduction of road traffic accidents involving children. These objectives probably cannot be reached using communicative interventions alone. We need legislation regarding speed reduction in the given area, forcing traffic participants to drive within the speed limit. There are financial consequences resulting from this legislation: if a driver is caught, it will cost him or her money. In addition, traffic calming measures can be built into the road ('facilities' in Figure 8.3), making it unpleasant to drive fast. Parents in the neighbourhood can place signs along the road stating: 'If you slow down, you will save our children'. This is a form of social influence. As we have seen in section 3.7, social influence can have an external (compliance: conform to a norm if others are present) and internal (acceptance: internalising the norm) influence on individual behaviour. In addition, communication, either about the importance of changing driving behaviour and/or the necessity of the measures taken, and the expected and obtained results (i.e. feedback) can complete the programme.

Developing communicative interventions
There is no simple answer to the question of how to design communicative interventions. The contents have to reflect the objectives to be achieved, adjusted to the characteristics of target group

(e.g. frame of reference). For the selection of message contents and communication methods, see Chapters 5 and 6. Previous research findings, lessons learned from other programmes, and earlier experience with activities on related issues might also be helpful. In the development of activities, it is important to link new activities to already existing activities and programmes. Therefore, it is important to create an overview of existing and available resources, existing examples of good practice, potential for change, and opportunities for action. Consideration is needed too about how to increase the chances of target groups being exposed to the intervention; this means that the selection of places in which information or instruction is provided is important. Criteria to scrutinise are attraction, attention, understanding, personal relevance, credibility, and acceptability of the communicative intervention.

Based on the selection of instruments, communication methods, and settings, the *programme objectives* need to be formulated. Programme objectives describe the specific activities that will be conducted in order to achieve the intervention objectives. They refer to message contents, communication methods, strategies and channels to be used, and settings in which the action takes place. The activities in the programme development phase are summarised in Table 8.4.

8.3.3 Assessment of resources and organisation

Identification of resources needs specific attention in programme development (*cf.* Boonekamp *et al.*, 1995). It is necessary to know which resources are available and under what conditions, which resources need to be acquired, and how such resources can be mobilised and organised. Resources are all the goods, funds, services, manpower, technology, material and equipment that are available to organise and carry out the programme and its activities in order to achieve the objectives. The financial aspect of the programme is a prime consideration. We must account for money not only to produce materials and for logistics, but also for the time people spend in production and implementation of the programme. Time is usually one of the biggest constraints in the implementation of a programme.

Table 8.4 *Summary of phases, activities, and objectives.*

Phase	Activities	Objectives
Diagnosis of existing situation	• assessment of perceived needs and priorities • examination of epidemiological data and social indicators • setting priorities for action	→ Health objectives –
Diagnosis of behavioural causes	• analysis of behavioural links with health problem • ratings of importance and changeability	→ Behavioural objectives
Diagnosis of environmental causes	• analysis of environmental links with the health problem • ratings of importance and changeability	→ Environmental objectives
Diagnosis of behavioural and environmental determinants	• analysis of determinants of behaviour in terms of its predisposing, reinforcing and enabling factors • analysis of environmental determinants • setting priorities	→ Intervention objectives • cognitive and psychomotoric • environmental conditions
Programme development	• building or extending networks for action • selection of instruments for changes in the environment • selection of message content, communication methods and settings	→ Programme objectives

→ objectives to be formulated

8.3.4 Formulation of programme plans

Once the programme team has discussed all the aspects of the plan, a written version should be prepared. This plan serves several purposes (Boonekamp *et al.*, 1995). Firstly, for the writing of the plan, ideas and procedures need to be clearly defined. Often the plan in one's mind is not as clear as one had thought, and the gaps and flaws are easier to recognise and to correct when it is written down on paper. As such, it illustrates contingency between the different parts of the programme. Secondly, it functions as a tool for participants to know what has to be done, by whom, and at what time, and it illustrates that concrete actions are part of a continuous programme. Thirdly, it constitutes a framework for monitoring and evaluation. Through monitoring it can be determined whether or not the plan is still adequate and whether things are proceeding as planned. In addition, it allows the programme to be studied and checked by anyone whose advice is desired, or whose support for the programme is required. The action plan should be agreed upon by all participants and provide an overview of:
- objectives, target groups, and activities;
- the roles and responsibilities of the participants;
- a timetable of events, including milestones and progress reports; and
- an overview of finances.

We want to point out, however, that programmes should not be too rigid. Some flexibility is needed. The programme has to be able to adapt to unforeseen changes while it is running, and to the reactions and emerging needs of the target group in particular. Agreements should be reached on procedures to be followed if additional decisions have to be made. This facilitates regular adjustments of the plan to changing circumstances or to new information.

So far, we have discussed programme development from a static perspective and have said that everything can be decided upon beforehand. In health promotion however, we often deal with situations in which interventions are *not* described in detail beforehand but are developed throughout the time the programme is running. This means that, even though in many programmes the subject is decided upon, including initial activities, not all interventions can be described carefully at the outset. New activities are often developed throughout the process of collective action, together with the people and organisations involved. According to Frankish and Green (1994), this increases the feelings of ownership and, in turn, ownership increases capacity (competence) and promotes programme maintenance. Of course, those interventions also need a plan for implementation.

Assessment of resources and the establishment of a plan for organisation are defined in the final set of objectives, the so-called process objectives. Process objectives refer to the organisation of the programme and resources necessary to implement the programme. They are formulated in terms of human and financial resources, as well as the division of roles and responsibilities of the participants in the programme, and they include a timescale. We summarise the activities again in Table 8.5.

8.3.5 Evaluability assessment

Before actual implementation, and as a final part of the programme development phase, comes evaluability assessment. Evaluability assessment can be considered as a kind of 'pre-evaluation' (Rossi & Freeman, 1993). It links the objectives that have been formulated at an earlier stage to both the programme that has been designed and the implementation plan. This type of evaluation is often conducted when the programme is running. We propose, however, to consider the important questions in the planning phase. The first important question is whether the chosen methods are appropriate for achieving the objectives as formulated. For example, if the objective is that 30 per cent of the defined population has the skills to increase physical exercise, and the programme organisers decide to address this issue only by means of a mass media campaign, it is to be expected that the objective will not be met. A consequence could be that the initial plans need to be revised or elaborated. Another consequence might be that the objectives have to be reformulated in such a way that they can actually be achieved given the planned activities. The second important issue concerns the feasibility of the programme. Can the programme be implemented as planned given the available resources in terms of time, manpower, materials and finances? Can the participants in the programme indeed play the role they are expected to play or the role they initially intended to play? If not, can additional resources be made available? These questions may lead to the conclusion that the plans are too ambitious and that the programme needs to be modified. The rationale for evaluability assessment in the planning phase is clear: it

Table 8.5 Summary of phases, activities, and objectives.

Phase	Activities	Objectives
Diagnosis of existing situation	• assessment of perceived needs and priorities • examination of epidemiological data and social indicators • setting priorities for action	→ Health objectives
Diagnosis of behavioural causes	• analysis of behavioural links with health problem • ratings of importance and changeability	→ Behavioural objectives
Diagnosis of environmental causes	• analysis of environmental links with the health problem • ratings of importance and changeability	→ Environmental objectives

Diagnosis of behavioural and environmental determinants	• analysis of determinants of behaviour in terms of its predisposing, reinforcing and enabling factors
	• analysis of environmental determinants
	• setting priorities
		→ Intervention objectives
		  • cognitive and psychomotoric
		  • environmental conditions

Programme development	• building or extending networks for action • selection of instruments for changes in the environment • selection of message content, communication methods and settings	→ Programme objectives
	• assessment of resources and organisation • formulation of the programme plan	→ Process objectives

→ objectives to be formulated

is wiser to make modifications prior to implementation than when the programme is already running. It facilitates a synthesis between intervention objectives, activities and programme objectives. Moreover, it increases the measurability of the outcomes of the programme, avoids disappointments, and increases the probability that the programme will indeed be effective.

8.4 Implementation

Once a programme has been developed, it is ready to be implemented. Implementation actually turns ideas and plans into action. Implementation, however, is not an autonomous, self-generating and self-perpetuating process. Programmes are often not implemented exactly the way they were planned. Several unanticipated difficulties may occur, such as delays in delivery of educational materials, failure to attract the target group's attention, or difficulties in the process of intersectoral collaboration and community participation. While the action plan is being put into practice, the people and teams responsible should keep in touch with what is going on. Continuous evaluation of the process and the activities is necessary, including programme coverage, and the short-term impact of (parts of) the programme. We refer to this as monitoring the programme. Successful implementation largely depends on good programme management, on clear communication structures between participants, and flexibility in the face of changing circumstances (see, for example, Green & Kreuter, 1991; Bracht *et al.*, 1999; Rossi & Freeman, 1993; Koelen & Vaandrager, 1995; Contu & Congiu, 1995; Koelen *et al.*, 2001).

Monitoring is essential for 'single action programmes', for example, a mass media campaign on safe sex, as well as for 'sequential, combined action programmes', such as most community-based projects. Decisions can be made as to whether or not a programme needs to be adapted based on information provided by monitoring. The sooner insight into these issues is available, the better and more effective the programme or project will be in the end. Moreover, results from monitoring are important for evaluation purposes. The word 'evaluation' is associated with the question '*did* the programme work?' referring to the extent to which the programme was able to achieve the objectives as formulated in the diagnosis and planning phase. But evaluation is more than this.

An equally important evaluation question is *why* the programme did or did not work. Therefore, monitoring is important. Waiting until the project has finished might lead to reconstructing situations and in this way a lot of valuable information may be lost (Koelen & Vaandrager, 1999). Information obtained through monitoring helps to understand the results as obtained in evaluation. We will deal with monitoring in detail in the next chapter.

Monitoring the programme during implementation aims to assess the extent to which the process and programme objectives have been achieved. To summarise the implementation phase, we extend our overview table further (Table 8.6).

Table 8.6 Summary of phases, activities, and objectives.

Phase	Activities	Objectives
Diagnosis of existing situation	• assessment of perceived needs and priorities • examination of epidemiological data and social indicators • setting priorities for action	→ Health objectives
Diagnosis of behavioural causes	• analysis of behavioural links with health problem • ratings of importance and changeability	→ Behavioural objectives
Diagnosis of environmental causes	• analysis of environmental links with the health problem • ratings of importance and changeability	→ Environmental objectives
Diagnosis of behavioural and environmental determinants	• analysis of determinants of behaviour in terms of its predisposing, reinforcing and enabling factors • analysis of environmental determinants • setting priorities	→ Intervention objectives • cognitive and psychomotoric • environmental conditions

Table 8.6 Continued.

Programme development	• building or extending networks for action • selection of instruments for changes in the environment • selection of message content, communication methods and settings	→ Programme objectives
	• assessment of resources and organisation • formulation of the programme plan	→ Process objectives
Implementation	• examination of organisational aspects, including • assessment of processes of participation and collaboration • examination of programme inputs	← Process objectives
	• assessment of unanticipated difficulties and side effects • monitoring of activities • short term impact	← Programme objectives

→ objectives to be formulated
← objectives to be evaluated

8.5 Evaluation

Evaluation to some extent takes place throughout the whole process, but specifically in the phase of implementation and evaluation. In the implementation phase, we refer to it as monitoring (or process evaluation). In the evaluation phase, the programme as a whole is considered. We distinguish between effectiveness, efficiency and validity evaluation. Effectiveness, efficiency and validity are related concepts insofar as they are all concerned with the achievement of health education and health promotion programmes. They differ in scope however. *Effectiveness* or outcome evaluation refers to the extent to which a programme has achieved its objectives, i.e. an evaluation of the intervention objectives. To recall, these are the objectives in which the expected change in cognitive, psychomotor, and environmental determinants of behaviour are expressed. *Efficiency* evaluation focuses on the achievement of behavioural and environmental objectives. In fact, it is a measure of relative effectiveness, that is, the extent to which a given programme has achieved its goals in comparison with alternative or competing interventions. For example, we can compare the results of a peer-led smoking reduction programme with the results of an expert-led one. If the peer-led programme leads to a more substantial decrease in the number of youngsters taking up smoking than the one that is expert-led, the peer-led programme is more efficient. Efficiency evaluation also includes the cost-effectiveness of competing programmes. Cost-benefit analysis tries to state both the costs and the benefits in monetary terms. Clearly, the benefits of preventive action are mostly difficult to express. Despite this, several authors have made comprehensive calculations, and found interesting cost-benefit ratios, showing the financial benefit of health programmes. For an overview of economic evaluation approaches we refer to Godfrey, 2001. Economic indicators should, however, be treated with caution. Health education and health promotion strive to add healthy years to life and to enhance the quality of that life. These values are hard to express in monetary terms. The third level of evaluation is validity evaluation. *Validity evaluation* focuses on the question of whether or not behavioural and environmental changes contribute to the achievement of the higher-level health objectives. The health objectives tend to be ambitious and broad. As mentioned previously, they are usually formulated in vague terms and do not provide clear criteria for evaluation. In spite of this, it is important to consider the achievements of a programme in the light of these long-term aims and objectives. Evaluation thus not only provides evidence as to *how* successful the programme has been, but also informs us as to *why* the programme was successful. As such, it provides a basis for decisions about future planning and programming. In the next chapter we will address the issue of evaluation in more detail.

The evaluation phase is summarised in Table 8.7, the final table. The table summarises each phase identified in the process of designing health education and health promotion programmes.

Table 8.7 Summary of phases, activities, and objectives.

Phase	Activities	Objectives
Diagnosis of existing situation	• assessment of perceived needs and priorities • examination of epidemiological data and social indicators • setting priorities for action	→ Health objectives
Diagnosis of behavioural causes	• analysis of behavioural links with health problem • ratings of importance and changeability	→ Behavioural objectives
Diagnosis of environmental causes	• analysis of environmental links with the health problem • ratings of importance and changeability	→ Environmental objectives

Diagnosis of behavioural and environmental determinants	• analysis of determinants of behaviour in terms of its predisposing, reinforcing and enabling factors
	• analysis of environmental determinants
	• setting priorities
		→ Intervention objectives
		  • cognitive and psychomotoric
		  • environmental conditions

Programme development	• building or extending networks for action • selection of instruments for changes in the environment • selection of message content, communication methods and settings	→ Programme objectives
	• assessment of resources and organisation • formulation of the programme plan	→ Process objectives

Table 8.7 Continued.

Implementation	• examination of organisational aspects, including	← Process objectives
	• assessment of processes of participation and collaboration	
	• examination of programme inputs	
	• assessment of unanticipated difficulties and side effects	← Programme objectives
	• monitoring of activities	
	• short term impact	
Evaluation	• effectiveness evaluation	← Intervention objectives
	• efficiency evaluation	← Behavioural and environmental objectives
	• validity evaluation	← Health objectives

→ objectives to be formulated
← objectives to be evaluated

8.6 Chapter summary

In this chapter we have given an overview of the different steps to be taken in the design and evaluation of effective health education and health promotion programmes. We identified four phases overall: diagnosis, programme development, implementation, and evaluation, and presented a hierarchy of objectives to be formulated and evaluated in the programme. In the diagnosis phase, problems and needs are identified, and analysed in terms of their behavioural and environmental causes and their determinants. The analysis generates health, behavioural, environmental, and intervention objectives. The programme development phase focuses on building networks for action, and on analysis of possibilities for action. Decisions are formulated in programme and process objectives. In the implementation phase, the planned programme is put into practice. Evaluation, mentioned as the fourth phase, is actually pivotal in each phase, but particularly in establishing whether or not the objectives have been achieved as set out during diagnosis. It should be noted that each phase in the process needs research. This will be addressed in the next chapter.

9. Research in health promotion

In the previous chapter we dealt with the design of health promotion programmes. We identified four phases: diagnosis, programme development, implementation and evaluation. Related to these phases we also distinguish between four phases in research: preliminary research, programme development research, monitoring, and evaluation. *Preliminary research* focuses on diagnosis of the existing situation, the environmental and behavioural causes of health problems and the determinants of these causes. *Programme development research* facilitates the development of programmes and action plans. *Monitoring* aims to examine the ways in which programmes are implemented, including the processes of participation and collaboration, in order to keep track of and/or improve the programme. *Evaluation* involves a review of the results achieved in the programme in terms of its effectiveness, efficiency and validity.

In health promotion there is a strong connection between action and research. Research facilitates practice in decisions that need to be made in order to run a programme, whereas practice simultaneously evokes questions that are relevant for research. Action and research in health promotion are therefore not separate activities, but are interrelated. The research itself can be considered part of the change process. The interrelation between research and action is illustrated in Figure 9.1.

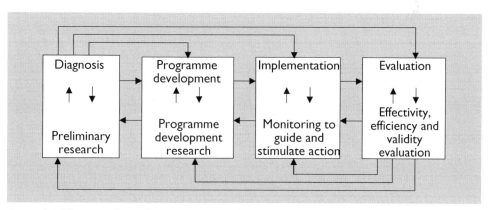

Figure 9.1 The interrelation between action and research.

In this chapter we firstly expatiate on different approaches to research, and we argue that health promotion needs an eclectic approach towards research methodologies. Next we discuss research in relation to the phases in the process of planning and evaluation. We address research in relation to diagnosis and programme development only briefly, but elaborate extensively on research in the implementation and evaluation phase. Research in these phases aims to show that health education and health promotion can be successful. Such data facilitate communication about the programme, both to the people who are directly involved and to other important individuals, such as policy makers and funding agencies.

9.1 Research typology

Health promotion is typically an eclectic field. New insights and theories are developed within the specific domain, but often theories and insights from other disciplines are applied, such as from psychology, sociology, marketing, management, communication, and economics. Using theories that transcend a domain-specific scope creates a far richer picture of the mechanisms of reality than a single domain can ever create. Along the same lines, we argue that using different approaches to research and a variety of research methodologies fosters both the practical and scientific development of the field. We briefly discuss some typologies of research, relating to the type of data, research styles, and to the research approach, which in our opinion are important.

9.1.1 Quantitative and qualitative research

Quantitative research collects data that can be expressed in numerical representations (quantity, amount, intensity, frequency) and that lend themselves to tests of statistical significance - for example, answers on structured questionnaires, counts of the incidence of certain behaviours, or counts of the number of interactions between certain groups. *Qualitative* research gathers data that can less easily, if at all, be expressed in meaningful numbers. This includes data such as the protocols of unstructured interviews, notes from observations, or minutes of meetings. Quantitative research focuses on the measurement and analysis of causal relations between variables. Qualitative research focuses on processes and meanings.

9.1.2 Research styles

In general, four styles of enquiry can be distinguished: experimental research, surveys, documentary-historical research, and field research (*cf.* Miller & Crabtree, 1992). *Experimental research* aims to study causal relations between two or more variables in tightly controlled conditions (usually in laboratory settings). The variable of interest, the independent variable, is carefully manipulated and its effect is measured on a pre-determined dependent variable. Take, for example, the hypothesis 'messages containing new arguments about an issue will lead to opinion change, whereas messages containing familiar arguments will not lead to opinion change'. In this example, the independent variable is the type of message, i.e. the extent to which the arguments provided are new or familiar. Opinion change is the dependent variable. To test this hypothesis, half the subjects in a study are exposed to new arguments and the other half to familiar arguments. The dependent variable is measured both before and after exposure to the message. If differences in opinion are found between pre- and post-test, then the type of message has caused this. In experimental research, measurements are quantitative in nature and results are expressed in terms of statistical significance. Experimental researchers aim to develop theories. They are generally not interested in either the societal or the practical relevance of the research results. For example, a researcher may study the influence of cholesterol on the development of cardiovascular disease, without being interested in its meaning for interventions.

Survey research aims at a description of real life phenomena in terms of their content and extent. Validated instruments are used for measurement, such as a structured interview, a rating scale, or a questionnaire. Data are gathered from a representative sample of the whole population, and it is expected that the results obtained from the sample can be generalised to apply to the larger population from which the sample was drawn. A research question could be for instance 'what is the current attitude of the population towards safer sex?' As with experimental research, data gathered are quantitative in nature, and differences are expressed in terms of statistical significance.

Documentary-historical inquiries focus on artefacts, such as archives, literature, medical records and minutes of meetings. Literature reviews and archive analysis as well as secondary analysis and meta-analysis are examples. For example, a content analysis may be conducted on the minutes of meetings of a programme team in order to analyse the historical development of community participation in the programme. The methods used can be both quantitative and qualitative.

In *field research* the focus is on generating realistic descriptions and explanations of a specified situation. Research questions immediately arise from the situation in hand. Research focuses on finding concrete solutions for concrete problems, resulting from concrete practice. Field research often takes the form of a case study or of a topical study. A case may be an individual, a specific setting such as a school, or a community. For example, in a certain area of a specific city, high crime rates are found. The question then is 'how can we effectively reduce crime and violence in this area?' Topical studies investigate only one or two selected issues, for example, a study of the meaning of following certain dietary guidelines for diabetes II patients. The methods used may be quantitative, but are often qualitative in nature.

9.1.3 Research approach

With regard to the research approach, a distinction can be made between 'traditional research' and 'action research'. In the *traditional research approach*, also referred to as the biomedical approach in the field of health, the researcher takes on the role of an external observer. Traditional research is based on the wish to discover, predict and control phenomena, and is typically related to experimental and survey research. Results from research are used 'to show', for instance to illustrate the complexity of a situation, to find support for a hypothesis, or to show whether or not an intervention is effective. The researcher takes away the information from the situation under study, and the results are presented after the research is complete. Action research is different. *Action research* focuses on a specific situation, and the results are used for decision making *in* that situation. Research aims to analyse a situation and its problems, to find solutions to address these problems, and to look at possibilities for putting these solutions into practice (Whyte *et al*, 1991). Results are thus immediately fed back into a programme. They are the point of departure for the people working in that practice and help them to decide how to continue. This research therefore literally aims to stimulate and guide action. A special form of action research is *participatory action research*. This is research in which the researcher collaborates with all the others involved, including members of the target groups. Participatory action research serves two functions: (a) a research function, to show processes, progress and results, and (b) an action function, i.e. a tool for action, reflection, discussion and decision making. It is essential that the results of each research step be fed back into the project immediately. In our opinion, participatory action research is of special relevance to health promotion. Participation in research by all stakeholders creates the opportunity to benefit from the knowledge by experience of target populations, and to obtain active support for the results of the process of inquiry. It facilitates commitment to change, and increases the likelihood that ideas and activities will be diffused. Participatory action research can thus be seen as an integral part of the change process.

9.1.4 The need for combined techniques

Health promotion research functions not only as a tool to *measure* change and innovation, but also as a tool to *facilitate* these outcomes. In our opinion, research needs to be methodologically eclectic. The above-described styles and approaches are equally important. They are not mutually exclusive and, in reality, the differences are often only slight. In fact, they need each other. Experimental research builds theories that are of great importance for practice. As Lewin stated: 'nothing is as practical as a good theory'. Questions for experimental research, however, often arise from practice, because, for instance, gaps in a theory become apparent in its application, or because of new discoveries that cannot be explained by the available theories. Different kinds of research can take place within one programme. Each of the abovementioned research styles and approaches may give limited insight when used alone, but the combination gives a rich picture of processes and achievements. An eclectic approach to research makes relevant contributions to both practice and science, and thereby to the development of a comprehensive theoretical basis for health promotion.

In the remainder of this chapter, we elaborate on research relating to the phases in the design and evaluation of health promotion programmes. The focus will be on ways of collecting information, in which we advocate the eclectic approach towards research.

9.2 Preliminary and programme development research

Preliminary research is carried out in the diagnosis phase and aims to get an understanding of the situation in hand. It includes assessment of behavioural and environmental factors contributing to identified health problems, and the identification of relevant stakeholders. At the individual level, information needs to be gathered about existing behaviour and lifestyle, and the related predisposing, reinforcing and enabling factors. Programme development research focuses on the collaboration and participation structure, the selection of intervention instruments, messages, communication methods, settings, and on the development of concrete action plans. Several research techniques may be used to gather the necessary information, for example:

- Epidemiological data, information regarding social indicators (e.g. unemployment, education) and demographic information can all be obtained by means of surveys. These data are often already archived however.
- Formal and informal interviews with key informants, such as community care centres, health professionals, representatives from community groups, school governors and/or teachers, and policy makers.
- Group sessions, using the nominal group process method. As this is a small group technique, it is particularly helpful in identifying and ranking (community) problems. This method is well described by Green and Kreuter (1991).
- Focus group interviews may be valuable for identifying and prioritising problems, as well as for finding possible solutions to these problems. Focus group interviews may be held with representatives from all groups relevant to the problem (e.g. health professionals, school teachers, community members). Such interviews are useful in each phase of the programme, i.e. in diagnosis, planning, implementation, and evaluation. Krueger (1991) provides an extensive description of this method.
- To obtain information about individual behaviour and the determinants of that behaviour, questionnaires may be administered

to a random sample of the population. The questionnaires can be developed, based on theories as described in Chapter 3, but one can also use questionnaires that have been developed and validated in other research. A helpful guide for the development of questionnaires can be found in Schwarz (1996). The results of such a survey can be used as baseline data for effectiveness evaluation at the individual level. In these cases, the same instrument is administered to the same sample both before (pre-test) and after (post-test) the programme is implemented

- The rapid participatory appraisal technique is helpful in order to obtain information about the structure of a community, as well as to identify relevant groups and organisations. Information is gathered in workshops with key informants and focuses on local knowledge. This technique enables a lot of qualitative data to be obtained about perceived problems as well as about the people and organisations involved in certain issues. Good descriptions as to how this method may be used are given by WHO (1991), Kumar (1993) and Grandstaff and Messerschmidt (1995).
- Several other research instruments are available for the identification of individuals or groups. In our research, instruments such as the stakeholder interest matrix and the stakeholder importance matrix (Groot, 1999) have proven to be adequate. These instruments provide information about sectors relating to a health problem, networking experience, the possible contribution of stakeholders and their possible role and function, mutual expectations and conditions for participation.

The information gathered in preliminary and programme development research forms the basis to set priorities and to formulate SMART objectives (see section 8.1). Moreover, information from preliminary research can be considered as baseline data against which the performance of a programme can be measured.

9.3 Monitoring

The importance of research during the implementation of health education and health promotion programmes is increasingly emphasised. The rationale is fourfold. *Firstly*, day-to-day monitoring is important in order to manage and administer the programme properly.

It helps to identify problems and unforeseen difficulties as well as providing information as to whether or not the programme is being implemented in compliance with its design, and whether or not it is reaching its specified target groups. Research in the implementation phase is often referred to as 'formative evaluation'. We prefer to use the term 'monitoring' however. The term is derived from the Latin word 'to warn', which is indeed one of its main functions. Early detection of problems enables one to adjust the programme, and thereby increases its chance of being effective. *Secondly*, insight into the implementation process enables the results of the outcome evaluation to be interpreted effectively. As Rossi and Freeman (1993:36) state, 'there is no point in being concerned with the impact or outcome of a particular project unless it has indeed taken place and served the appropriate participants in the way intended'. Monitoring reduces the risk of a Type III error, i.e. a conclusion that a campaign is ineffective when in fact the campaign was not implemented as designed. (Note that a Type I error refers to the conclusion that a campaign was effective when in fact it was not; a Type II error refers to the conclusion that a campaign was not effective when in fact it was.) *Thirdly*, health promotion programmes usually start as temporary projects, but the intention is that they become sustainable. Therefore, special attention is necessary for the integration of intervention activities into community networks (Bracht *et al.*, 1999). Monitoring can provide information about the processes of achieving and sustaining collective action. It helps to find solutions while working together with those involved in the programme. It offers the opportunity for 'learning by doing'. *Finally*, monitoring provides information that helps to pinpoint why a given programme succeeded or failed, which is important for decisions about possible continuation of the programme, or for possible relocation to other sites, other groups, and other settings.

Monitoring can be considered as research to guide and stimulate action. With reference to the hierarchy of objectives as presented in section 8.1, monitoring focuses on the extent to which the process and programme objectives are achieved. These are the objectives in which the programme and the requirements to successfully run the programme are described. Monitoring focuses on both implementation of the programme activities and the processes of intersectoral collaboration and community participation. We will deal with them separately.

9.3.1 Research to monitor the programme

The impact of a programme can be sharply diminished and sometimes even reduced to zero when it is not appropriately delivered. Monitoring is an instrument to help to overcome such problems. Programme monitoring is generally defined as the systematic examination of programme coverage and delivery (Rossi & Freeman, 1993). It provides information about inputs, organisational aspects, coverage and short-term effectiveness. Insight into these aspects enables us to see whether the programme is running as planned and whether adjustment of activities is necessary.

- *Examination of the programme inputs* includes assessment of the allocated and expended resources in terms of time, staff, money, accommodation and materials. All these inputs can be recorded during implementation. Measuring the inputs is necessary to be able to make judgements about whether the outcome was worthwhile.
- *Examination of organisational aspects* refers to questions such as: is the programme being implemented in the ways envisaged, are the activities being conducted as planned, did the materials arrive at the right time and at the right place, are the materials being used as intended, are the resources and means sufficient, is the intended manpower available and sufficient?
- *Programme coverage* refers to the reach of the activities, more specifically, to the extent to which the target groups are exposed to the programme. Important questions are: are the members of the target group aware of and familiar with the activities, do they receive the materials as planned, and do they participate in activities, both as 'consumers of the activities' and as 'partners in action? A typical challenge for programme planners is to attract attention to its activities. Attracting interest for a programme or parts of it is a precondition for success. Additional questions relate to appreciation of the activities, and the short-term impact, that is, whether the programme is able to cause change in the desired direction.
- *Examination of unanticipated side effects* includes both positive and negative side effects. For instance, during a stop-smoking programme, people who give up cigarettes might decide to increase physical exercise, but they might also replace cigarettes with large amounts of sweets.
- *Examination of events not related to the intervention*: During the course of a programme, events may occur that are not related to the

intervention, but which influence its impact. For example, a government decision to increase tax on alcoholic beverages during a campaign to reduce alcohol consumption probably affects drinking behaviour. In this example, the event will strengthen the impact of the campaign, but events can also reduce the impact. For example, a report in the newspaper that people with low cholesterol levels are more prone to depression may cause the message 'reduce cholesterol intake' to be ignored.

Data for monitoring may be collected in many different ways - for example, direct observation during activities, focus group interviews with those who take part in the activities, and interviews (oral, telephone, written questionnaire) with conductors of the programme. In addition, records may be kept regarding the number and type of activities conducted, the number and type of participants involved in the activities, the number and type of contributors to the activities and the costs involved in the activities. This may become part of a systematic management information system. Minutes of planning meetings can also be used for monitoring.

9.3.2 Research to monitor the processes of participation and collaboration

Intersectoral collaboration and community participation are important processes in health promotion, but they are also difficult to achieve and to sustain. Regular assessment of how these processes function in practice, and discussion among the participants about their experiences of collective action, can facilitate and support the process. Assessment of these processes has a double function: (1) to evaluate the state of the art, and (2) to enable the participants to identify elements for improvement. Collaboration and participation can be assessed with the help of both quantitative and qualitative indicators. Examples of quantitative indicators are summarised in Table 9.1.

Quantitative data, however, do not provide a measure of the *quality* of participation and collaboration. Quality refers to the level of satisfaction with the functioning of the network, and includes such aspects as influence on decisions, the quality of the decisions, and satisfaction with the role and responsibilities of oneself and of the others in the network. Rifkin has developed a useful instrument to assess this

Table 9.1 Quantitative indicators to assess intersectoral action.

- Count of opportunities to set up common activities
- Percentage of inhabitants that participate in the planning and implementation of activities
- Numbers of collaboration structures, members, member growth and member decrease
- Frequency of meetings
- Number of stakeholders attending planned meetings
- Number of contacts between the groups involved, both within and outside the programme
- Number of tasks of each participant in the programme
- Time spend on the programme by the participants

quality, the so-called participation measurement instrument (Rifkin *et al.*, 1988; Rifkin, 2000). This instrument assesses the functioning of a network in relation to needs assessment, leadership, organisation, resource mobilisation, and management. In our research (e.g. Koelen & Vaandrager, 1995), we combined this instrument with Pretty's (1995) ladder of participation (see Table 7.1). This ladder identifies seven levels: no participation, passive participation, participation by information giving, participation by consultation, functional participation, interactive participation, and self-mobilisation. Participants in a programme are asked individually to respectively indicate which level according to their own perception (a) actually exists, (b) is considered desirable, and (c) is achievable. The individual scores are summarised and fed back into the groups that provided the information. Reflection and discussion of results with the stakeholders illuminates the main problems and challenges, and enables participants to identify elements for improvement in future collaborations.

This instrument can be used at several points throughout a project. In this way, it serves a twofold function. Firstly, it evaluates the state of the art of the networks as well as visualising changes in the quality of participation in time, thus serving an evaluation function. Secondly, it facilitates discussion about the processes, enabling participants to identify elements for improvement in future collaborations.

9.4 Evaluation research

Evaluation research is usually considered to be the final part of a programme, but evaluation requires input from the very beginning. Preliminary research offers the baseline information against which the results of the final evaluation can be compared. Programme development research leads to feasible programmes. Monitoring provides information about the extent to which the programme was able to induce any change. Hence, each phase provides information necessary for the interpretation of the results.

Evaluation research is important for several reasons. *Practice* benefits from knowledge about the extent to which objectives are achieved, and insight into the strong and weak points of the programme and its parts. This information is necessary not only for quality improvement, but also for decisions relating to future planning. Results of evaluation may be decisive in 'go/no-go' decisions for future action. Evaluation research moreover serves *legitimation and accountability*. Planners and programme managers need to distinguish effective programmes from ineffective ones. Policy makers and funding agencies have a right to demand evidence that the money they spend is well spent. Finally, evaluation research contributes to the development of *scientific knowledge* and thereby to the development of theory.

9.4.1 Criteria for success

The main focus in evaluation is the question of the extent to which the programme has been successful in reaching its objectives. In discussing the formulation of objectives in the previous chapter, we presented a hierarchy of objectives. Health objectives, at the top of the hierarchy, are usually formulated in ambitious and broad terms. Further down the hierarchy, the objectives become more achievable and measurable, and achieving objectives down the hierarchy is conditional to the achievement of objectives further up. Therefore, criteria for success are not related to the final health objectives only. There are several intermediate indicators to be considered when examining the success of health promotion programmes: those criteria that have to be met in order to achieve the long-term outcomes. Along the same lines, Tones and Tilford (1994) argue that it is useful to think of a kind of 'proximal-distal' chain of interventions, thereby referring to the relationship between a succession of programme inputs and outcomes. Several authors argue that it is meaningful to develop a sequence of indicators (e.g. Tones & Tilford, 1994; Koepsell *et al.*, 1995; MacDonald & Davies, 1998; Nutbeam, 1998b; Koelen *et al.*, 2001; Goodstadt *et al.*, 2001). Different terminology is used for this, but we propose the following: proxy indicators, intermediate indicators, distal indicators, and final indicators. *Proxy indicators* relate to the inputs to the programme. They relate to what we call the process and programme objectives. Proxy indicators have to be measured during monitoring in the implementation phase (see 9.3.1). *Intermediate indicators* refer to the achievements in relation to the determinants of behaviour, such as awareness of the problem, knowledge and changes in beliefs and attitudes, and the environmental conditions. They thus relate to the intervention objectives. *Distal indicators* measure the outcomes at the level of specified behaviours, such as smoking, physical exercise, and wearing a helmet when cycling in traffic - indeed, the indicators that are defined in the behavioural and environmental objectives. *Final indicators* are those elements that have been defined in the health objectives. To summarise, on the way to meeting health objectives, there are several intermediate criteria that may provide an educated estimate of success.

9.5 Evaluation research in practice

Effectiveness evaluation determines whether or not a programme has been able to induce any change in individual members of the target groups. Moreover, effectiveness evaluation generally uses quantitative measurements (quantity, amount, frequencies), and the research style resembles experimental research or surveys. This is also the starting point for the following discussion. In section 9.5.3 we again take the broader approach.

In effectiveness evaluation, we look for a *causal relation* between the interventions and the observed outcomes. The extent to which we can make reliable statements about this causal relation depends on internal validity. *Internal validity* is defined as the extent to which the research design permits one to reach causal conclusions (Cook & Campbell, 1979). Research is internally valid when the causal relation between the independent variable (e.g. the intervention) and the dependent variable (e.g. increase in knowledge) as found in our research, is also existent in reality. In order to be able to make credible statements about the effectiveness of interventions, an adequate research design is necessary. A design is a guide which specifies for whom interventions will be implemented, and on whom and when measurements will be made. Selection of the research design needs careful consideration because it actually determines to a large extent the validity, credibility and confidentiality of the statements that can be made about the outcomes. In section 9.2 we mentioned that the results of a survey, conducted amongst a representative sample of the target population in preliminary research, could be used as baseline data (pre-test) for effectiveness evaluation if the same questionnaire is administered when the intervention programme is complete (post-test). The differences between the two tests are a measure of the impact of the programme. However, health education and health promotion are typically carried out in natural settings. In section 9.3 we mentioned that while the programme is running, several events might occur which do not belong to the actual intervention, but which have an influence on the dependent variables. Hence, such events can form a severe threat to internal validity. The question then is: how sure are we that observed changes have indeed been caused by the intervention? Were there other influences that actually caused the change? In the following section we describe some threats to internal validity that are likely to occur in health programmes, and then return to the question of what possibilities exist to control for such threats. This is strongly related to the design of the study.

9.5.1 Threats to internal validity

All source books about research and research designs deal with internal validity and threats to internal validity. Here, we describe some of the most common threats found in research in real life situations. The definitions are based on Cook and Campbell (1979:51-55).

- *History* refers to a situation in which an event takes place between pre-test and post-test that is not related to the intervention but influences the outcome measures - for example, a tax increase on tobacco products during a stop-smoking programme.
- *Maturation* is an effect that might occur due to the respondents' growing older, wiser, stronger, or more experienced between the pre-test and post-test, when this maturation is not the treatment of

research interest. Maturation is a threat that may typically occur in programmes aimed at children. Their natural growth in cognitive skills may affect the measurement of knowledge on certain topics.

- *Testing* is a threat to internal validity when an effect might be due to the number of times particular responses are measured. Familiarity with a test can enhance performance, because items are more likely to be remembered at later testing sessions. Also, the mere fact of being exposed to a test may have an influence. We observed this aspect of testing in a study on nutrition education in a supermarket. Prior to the activities, a short questionnaire was administered to a sample of shoppers about their food pattern and food buying behaviour. After the activities, the same respondents where again asked to fill in the questionnaire, as were a new sample group of shoppers. We found that those who were involved in the pre-test had seen more of the activities in the supermarket than those who only participated in the post-test.
- *Instrumentation* refers to a bias caused by a change in the measuring instrument, or in data collection procedures between the pre-test and post-test. For example, observers become more experienced between pre-test and post-test. Also, if scales with unequal intervals are used for measuring, this may constitute an instrumentation threat.
- *Selection* occurs if people in the intervention group differ from those in the control group against which the results are compared. For example, there may be a pre-existing difference in knowledge about a certain topic between both groups.
- *Mortality* refers to a bias that occurs when people drop out of a particular treatment group during the course of the intervention. For example, in nutrition education programmes, those who fail to follow the recommendations may drop out. As a consequence, the group at the post-test differs from the pre-test group.
- *Diffusion of treatments* occurs when interventions are diffused to the control group.

9.5.2 Selection of research designs

The design that will overcome most of the threats to internal validity is the randomised control trial (RCT), also known as the biomedical research design. In this design, respondents are randomly assigned to treatment groups, that is, to the experimental group (E: the group that is exposed to the treatment) or to a control group (C: the group that is not exposed to the treatment). Both groups receive a pre-test and a post-test (see Figure 9.2.a). Consider the example of an experiment in which new drugs are tested. After agreement on participation in the study between the researchers and the patients, and after the signing of an informed consent, patients are randomly assigned to the treatment group or to the placebo group. Random assignment creates groups that are similarly constituted on the average, which means that the effects of selection and maturation can be ruled out. Each group is exposed to the same testing conditions (no testing problems) and experiences the same global pattern of history. Moreover, if there are treatment-related differences in drop out, this may be interpreted as a consequence of the treatment. Thus, randomisation prevents most threats to internal validity (*cf.* Cook & Campbell, 1979; Judd *et al.*, 1991). Experimental designs offer the best possibilities for reaching valid and credible causal statements.

In practice, randomisation is often not feasible. For example, it may not be possible to randomly assign individual members of a community (e.g. geographical area, school, or workplace) to the intervention and others to the non-intervention situation. A potential alternative could be to include different areas in the study, where the areas are randomly assigned to one of the conditions. In practice however, this will not lead to comparison groups that are similarly constituted on the average. Different areas in the same city or areas in different cities, even though they seem comparable, often differ on important background variables.

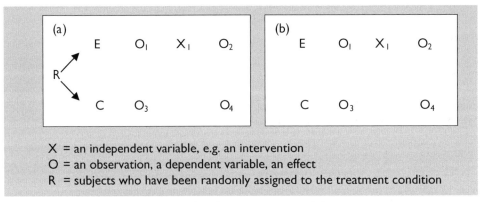

Figure 9.2 *Experimental and quasi-experimental design.*

In practice therefore, we usually have to rely on at best a *quasi-experimental design*. This design is similar to the experimental design, but individuals are not randomly assigned to one of the groups. Efforts need to be made to find groups that are more or less similar in important characteristics. For example, to study the effects of a nutrition education programme in schools, a control group may be found in another school serving the same age groups, standards and type of education. However, selection and history cannot be ruled out.

In health education and health promotion practice, it is often difficult to find adequate control groups. Programmes are carried out in field settings. These settings are generally open to the public at large, and people living in the control areas also have access to the programme. Moreover, mass media, such as local newspapers, radio and television programmes, may report the activities on several occasions. Hence, diffusion of the treatment to control groups is almost inevitable. Also, we often deal with so-called full-coverage programmes. For example, most campaigns sponsored by national governments aim to reach the whole population. Programmes in settings such as schools, the workplace, or hospitals aim to reach all members of the population. How then can we produce credible estimates of programme effectiveness? Two designs that are often applied in such situations are the one group pre-test/post-test design, and the time series design.

The *one group pre-test/post-test design* is based on 'within individual comparisons'. Participants in the study function as their own controls. This is also referred to as reflexive control. The design is schematically presented as:

Group 1 O_1 X O_2

Participants receive a pre-test prior to the programme, which is administered again after their exposure to the intervention. The impact of the intervention is estimated by examining the difference between O_2 and O_1. However, observed differences between before and after the intervention cannot be confidentially ascribed to the programme, since external influences cannot be disentangled from the influence of the intervention. Obviously, this design is not threatened by selection, but the threats of history, maturation, testing and instrumentation cannot be ruled out.

The time series design is an extension of the one group pre-test/post-test design. In fact, adding a number of pre-test and post-test measurements extends the design. It is schematically presented as follows:

Group 1 O_1 O_2 O_3 O_4 X O_5 O_6 O_7 O_8

The design thus involves repeated measurements of the same group of people over a period of time, both before and after the intervention. From the point of view of internal validity, this design is substantially stronger. The additional measures can help to control for the internal validity threats of maturation, testing and history. Therefore, it can produce results with a higher degree of credibility than a design with single measurements. For instance, you run a programme in a school, aiming to increase students' participation in sports activities. A remarkable increase in sports participation is found between O_4 and O_5, and you wonder whether this difference can be considered to result from intervention X. The additional measurements allow for the inspection of all the intervals before and after the intervention in order to look for maturation trends. According to Judd *et al.* (1991) if maturation were taking place, it would show up as a long-term trend, producing similar differences between O_1 and O_2, between O_2 and O_3, and so on, along the entire series of measurements. If none of the intervals shows such a trend, and the only difference lies between O_4 and O5, maturation is not a plausible explanation. Similarly, examination of the preceding and succeeding intervals provides a fair estimate of the influence of testing and history.

The question as to which design is the best in a given situation is not easy. Due to the fact that many intervention programmes are conducted in natural settings, it is usually not possible to select the design that is 'scientifically best'. We often have to rely on incomplete designs because it is difficult or impossible to construct meaningful control groups. It is generally argued that incomplete designs provide weak evaluations of effectiveness, because it is not possible to take confounding effects into account. Even if the practical value of the results may be clear, statements of causality are impossible. Not surprisingly, it is also a topic of lengthy debate between scholars and practitioners. Some argue that the only acceptable method is the randomised controlled trial, whereas others argue that the nature of health promotion requires a variety of research approaches. We clearly belong to this latter group. In our opinion, it is possible to arrive at reliable and valid conclusions, even when randomised controlled trials appear to be inapplicable. Gathering data on several occasions, combined with sophisticated monitoring, allows a firm assessment of outcomes to be made. Here we return to our eclectic approach. Koelen *et al.* (2001) describe strategies that can be used to increase the credibility and validity of research results. These strategies are derived from experiences in community-based health promotion programmes.

9.5.3 Increasing credibility and validity of research in practice

A promising approach to improving confidence in research findings relates to the concept of triangulation. Triangulation simply means using more than one approach to answer the same question. It represents a crosschecking of information, using multiple sources, multiple methods and multiple investigators (Tashakkori & Teddlie, 1998; Gifford, 1996). The concept of *multiple sources* means using multiple copies of one source (for example, interviews with several members of one social group), or different sources concerning one issue (for example, interviews with consumers, health and welfare professionals and volunteers about perceived nutrition-related problems). Using *multiple methods* refers to the comparison of results derived from a range of methods - for example, comparing the results of observation in schools with the results of interviews with parents and group discussions with teachers. Once a proposition is confirmed by one or more methods, the uncertainty of its interpretation is greatly reduced. The idea of *multiple investigators* is especially strong in health promotion, particularly if a participatory research approach is adopted. With the variety of individuals and groups involved in community-based health promotion for instance, each brings in their own specific domain of knowledge and information, as well as their own vision and standards. Exchanges of ideas and debates about differences lead to sophisticated information and definition of the situation at hand and give insight into situations asking for improvement. When the participants agree on interpretations of results, the threat of biased interpretations is considerably reduced. Interpretations with a high level of agreement can be considered reliable, whereas disagreement should lead to further inquiry. Through triangulation, we thus combine information obtained from different quantitative and qualitative sources.

Another interesting approach is that of *participant check*. This involves the feedback of interpretations and conclusions drawn by researchers to the people with whom the original information was constructed. The objective is to test the data, interpretations and conclusions. If the reconstructions by the researchers are recognised by the participants as adequate representations of their own realities, the credibility of the findings is enhanced. Participant checks can be applied to different groups, for example during focus group sessions with members of the target groups, or in workshops with people who actively contribute to the programme. The methods we presented when we described the monitoring of intersectoral collaboration and community participation also make use of this strategy. The important element is that participants have the opportunity to hear a summary of what investigators have learned about and constructed with the information they have gathered, that they can scrutinise and challenge these findings, and that they can volunteer additional information.

Finally we wish to look at the idea of *multiple cases*, that is, parallel investigations in different settings. The multiple case approach is a sort of meta-analysis, that is, a set of (statistical) procedures designed to accumulate results across independent studies that address a related set of research questions. Multiple cases are essential, as they can demonstrate replication. Experience is affirmed if other research teams proceed with parallel investigations using similar techniques and come up with similar results. Conducting comparable studies in different situations makes it possible to draw conclusions not only about the quality of achievements and the processes in force in community-based projects, but also about the usefulness of (new) research techniques. This offers the potential to develop strategies that are useful in other communities. Multiple case studies provide a basis for generalising the results to other situations.

Strategies to increase the validity of research results are in fact essential parts of the working process of health promotion. They provide information about processes and effective elements of a programme at different levels: the individual level, the organisational level, and the environmental level. The practical relevance is therefore clear, but the steps are also a basis for scientific validation. They provide the criteria against which the information can be judged, much as statistical analyses provide grounds for judgement in conventional methods. It also shows the importance of an eclectic approach, that is, using a combination of quantitative and qualitative methods, different styles of enquiry and different approaches. Consistency in results obtained through this variety of methods provides sophisticated insight into the process of change in populations and organisations, and can provide powerful evidence of success. Moreover, using a participatory approach to research contributes to the empowerment of all stakeholders involved, thus also for the community participants. Participation is a fundamental element of empowerment. By participating, people learn skills and experience feelings of self-enhancement that they carry beyond the specific situation.

9.6 Chapter summary

In this chapter we have addressed the role of research in health education and health promotion. We briefly discussed some typologies of research and argued that research in the health field has to be methodologically eclectic. The remainder of the chapter has been devoted to research in relation to the phases in designing and evaluating health-improving programmes. A distinction was made between preliminary research, programme development research, monitoring, and evaluation. Several ways of collecting data were discussed. We described ways of monitoring the programme (systematic examination of programme coverage and delivery), and of assessing the processes of intersectoral collaboration and community participation. Special attention was given to evaluation research. We discussed threats to internal validity and to the selection of research designs. Since health education and health promotion are conducted in natural settings, it is often difficult to select the design that is 'scientifically best'. However, the use of a variety of research methods provides powerful evidence of success.

10. Organisation and management

The environment and conditions under which health organisations operate are continuously changing. Throughout the previous chapters, several of these changes have been described and discussed. Some of the major breakthroughs to be identified are:

- The growing recognition of the holistic view of health issues. It is becoming widely accepted that there are a variety of factors affecting health. This has consequences for what actions are considered appropriate in promoting the positive health of populations. These include disease prevention, health protection, and health promotion.
- The notion that positive health can only be achieved if changes occur at multiple social levels, including the individual, organisations, communities and, in fact, society as a whole. This points to the necessity of partnerships between governmental and non-governmental organisations at both national and local level, as well as between organisations and communities.
- Empowerment is becoming an increasingly important issue. This implies that there is a need to increase the ability of individuals and groups to express and to solve their own problems. Facilitation of decision-making processes and of building capacity for action is becoming an increasingly important task of health organisations. These issues are not easy to realise. Organisations are generally used to working *for*, as opposed to working *with*, groups, communities, or other parts of the population. Besides, the public are generally not used to being actively involved in programmes.
- Major issues of concern change continuously, due to new insights, knowledge, health hazards, and societal change. For instance today, issues such as obesity and the consequences of aging increasingly receive attention, whereas a few decades ago they were unimportant.
- The number of information sources is still growing. Developments in information and communication technologies have opened up many new opportunities for obtaining and transferring information. People only turn to professionals for information in those areas where they provide more relevant, more reliable and more timely information at a lower cost than other sources. Health promoting

organisations themselves should use all available new sources of information, including people's indigenous knowledge and experience.

- Many health-education and health-promotion practices are proven to be un-sustainable. The development of more sustainable practices often requires collective decision making, as opposed to 'individual organisation decisions'.
- The increasingly acknowledged relationship between the health of a population and environmental health. In today's society, there is an alarming tendency towards the diminution of natural resources and increasing problems with pollution and environmental damage. Thus, we need not only to protect populations from environmental hazards, but also to protect the environment from human hazards (Simnett, 1995:14).
- There are strong tendencies towards changes in the financing of health service organisations through privatisation and financial support of government to Non-Governmental Organisations.

Since organisations have to perform specific tasks in a changing society, the design of organisations also has to change. Health organisations need to consider the appropriateness of their organisation to anticipate the abovementioned changes. Changes are needed in the ways in which health professionals perform their tasks, as well as in their relations with target populations. Organisations have to work together to obtain better results. Managers need to be sensitive to these developments, because they will have an important task in guiding the change process. As Simnett (1995:13) states, learning how best to work together is probably the biggest challenge facing the management of health promotion activities. We cannot indicate clearly which changes are needed in a given situation, but we will discuss some principles in this chapter that may help organisations, their managers, and their staff members to guide these change processes.

In this chapter we firstly elaborate on organisations and their environment. We go on to discuss some of the important conditions for the functioning of organisations, with special emphasis on communication. Finally, we pay particular attention to the organisation and management of intersectoral health promotion projects.

10.1 The environment of organisations: an open systems theory

Organisations do not function in isolation, but are part of a larger social structure. Organisations are generally open to their environment and must achieve an appropriate relationship with that environment if they are to survive. Looking at organisations in this way is based on the so-called 'open systems approach' to organisations as developed by Von Bertalanffy (1962). The open systems approach focuses on some key issues. Firstly, there is an emphasis on the environment in which organisations perform. This means that a lot of attention has to be devoted to the immediate task-environment, as defined by the organisation's direct interactions (e.g. clients, suppliers, and governmental agencies), as well as to the broader contextual or general environment (Morgan, 1986). Secondly, the open systems approach defines an organisation in terms of subsystems and the interrelationships between them. Systems consist of individuals who belong to groups, who belong to departments, that belong to an organisation, that belongs to the wider context of (indeed) communities, that in turn are made up of a variety of other subsystems. Thirdly, the open systems approach attempts to establish congruencies between different systems, and to identify and eliminate potential dysfunctions. This refers to principles such as requisite variety, differentiation and integration for organising different kinds of tasks within the same organisation (Morgan, 1986). Organisations thus are systems in themselves, whilst at the same time they are subsystems of the larger environment, for instance the community.

Communities can be considered from an open systems perspective as well. It allows a better understanding of the relationships between the various community levels and sectors. Important subsystems of any community system include the political sector, economic sector, health sector, education sector, communication sector, religious sector, recreational sector, social welfare sector, voluntary and statutory groups, and other groups that may be specific to particular communities. In Figure 10.1 we illustrate the interrelation between several subsystems.

Organisations increasingly have to work together in order to achieve their own goals, and certainly in order to achieve goals at a higher level.

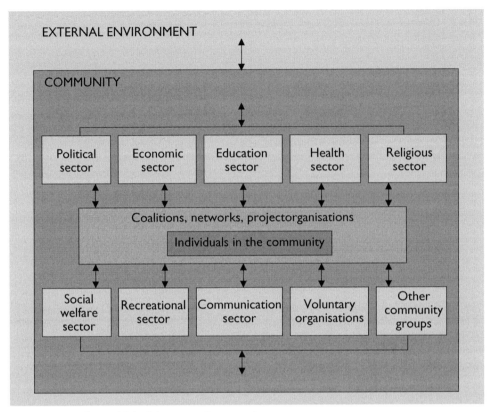

Figure 10.1 Schematic of community as an open system.

In fact, this relates to the key issue of health promotion. The overall aim of health promotion cannot be achieved by individual health organisations; neither can it be assured by the health sector alone. It demands, as stated by WHO (1986), an intersectoral approach and coordinated action from governments, health and other sectors, and from non-governmental and voluntary organisations. All of these organisations aim to produce their own goods or services. For example, schools provide education, hospitals provide treatment, the police provide safety and security, and cultural organisations provide leisure activities. When contributing to health promotion activities, organisations move to areas that are complementary to their main tasks - areas with which they are often not equipped to deal. Inducing changes in one sector or subsystem is not sufficient; a broader approach is needed in order to be successful in creating change in the community.

10.2 Factors influencing the functioning of organisations

Not all organisations involved in health promotion are health organisations. We can distinguish between organisations with a main role in the field of health, and organisations with a different main focus but contributing to the field of health, such as environmental health services, leisure services, the police force, the food industry, and schools. However, as Simnett (1995:14) states, to be successful we need organisations that aim to promote health *in* and *through* themselves; that is, organisations which improve health because of the intrinsic ways in which they set about their work, as well as through undertaking particular health promotion activities. This implies that organisations need to be sensitive to the health and wellbeing of all the people they work with and for, including management, employees, students, and customers (e.g. patients, consumers). The organisation of work, whether it is based in one organisation or in partnerships, requires certain conditions. We elaborate further on this subject in the following sections.

10.3 Networking and communication management

One important part of collaboration is networking. Networking is the creation of communication structures for the sharing of ideas, experience and information. Health promotion needs an interactive exchange of information. Communication management therefore is an essential task of any health organisation. Here we consider two distinct communication structures, namely external and internal communication.

10.3.1 External communication
External communication consists of two trajectories: the external-internal and internal-external communication trajectory. Both need considerable attention. For reasons of survival, competitive position, and finding out about possibilities for mutual gain in collaborations, it

is essential for any organisation to know the environment in which it functions. Organisations have to be alert to what is going on 'outside', they have to give information about themselves to that environment (the internal-external trajectory) and in addition they have to monitor and interpret outside information (the external-internal trajectory). However, the outside world is complex, and organisations have to deal with a variety of 'inputs'.

The external-internal trajectory

Van Woerkum *et al.* (1999) refer to 'conditional groups' and 'other input groups' on the *external-internal trajectory*. The *conditional groups* are groups that are conditional for the survival of an organisation in that they control the resources; that is, they provide organisations with a budget and manpower, which in turn influence their goals and those of the target populations they serve. In the commercial sector, this can be the parent organisation. In public health, this will often be a governmental organisation. For reasons of survival it is important to know the policy of the dominant organisation and to keep informed about statements of intent, in order to be able to anticipate decisions taken at a conditional level. The conditional groups are changing continuously, and the pace of this change is increasing. Hence, organisations need to be aware of these changes in time to make adjustments or, wherever possible, to participate in these changes.

The *other input groups* provide important inputs for the functioning of the organisation, such as knowledge, facilities or manpower. Consider, for instance, information on changes in the cultural interests of young people, or in the development of legislation relating to working conditions. In a sense, this also refers to the relation between professional organisations and research institutes. On the one hand, organisations and their staff responsible for developing health interventions must know the research findings that are relevant for their work. On the other hand, researchers should understand the problems and situations of the target populations in order to conduct research that delivers relevant information for health interventions. One difficulty is that researchers often gain greater rewards by undertaking research and producing articles that are published in scientific journals - thus earning them more recognition among other researchers - than they would gain from providing research findings that would help practitioners to work more effectively.

The internal-external trajectory

On the *internal-external trajectory,* Van Woerkum *et al.* (1999) describe 'output groups', 'groups serving common or related objectives', and 'normative relation groups'. *Output groups* are the consumers of the products or services the organisation supplies, such as customers, students, patients, or community members. For the survival of an organisation it is important to satisfy the needs of these consumers, and therefore it is important to know what they think, want and expect. *Groups serving common or related objectives* are mostly in competition. They strive for survival, sometimes at the expense of others- for instance, two regional schools each claiming to be the best in order to attract the most students. Sometimes organisations have to put substantial effort into transforming competitive relationships into collaborative ones if they need each other to achieve certain goals. The large number of organisations involved in health education and health promotion makes it difficult to develop an effective communication system. It is clear that communication with related groups is of special relevance. The third type of group is the *normative relation group.* These are groups that are in a position to influence the public image of an organisation by making value judgements about it, such as whether it is good or bad, traditional or innovative, whether or not it is credible, or whether or not it is consumer oriented. These groups therefore have an important influence on the image of the organisation. We can consider in this respect the mass media (e.g. newspapers, television, radio) or groups with strong media influence, such as consumer organisations, patient groups, political parties, religious organisations, or trade unions.

10.3.2 Internal communication

A good *internal communication structure* is one of the primary requirements in any organisation. Internal communication is the communication within the organisation or within a project. In section 9.5.3 we emphasised the importance of internal communication in increasing the credibility and validity of research results; but internal communication is also essential for keeping track of developments, for exchanging ideas and expectations, for receiving continued support, and to facilitate motivation. Katz and Kahn (1978) distinguish three internal information flows: downward communication, horizontal communication, and upward communication. The *downward communication* flow follows the hierarchical line of the organisation. It basically consists of specific job instructions, job rationale, organisational procedures and practices, feedback about performance, and information of an ideological nature in order to inculcate a sense of mission. The *horizontal communication* flow refers to communication among peers at the same organisational level. Its primary function is that of coordination of the work process between peers. In addition, it contributes to the mutual understanding of colleagues. It can provide both emotional and social support to the individual, and it offers an opportunity to learn from one another's experiences. *Upward communication* ascends the hierarchical structure. It relates to what people say about themselves, their performance, and their problems; about others and their performance and problems; about organisational practices and policies; and about what needs to be done and how it can be done.

Each internal flow of communication is important for any organisation. It should be noted that the length of each flow depends on the organisational structure. In highly bureaucratic organisations, the lines of communication are long; in adhocracies the lines are very short. According to Katz and Kahn (1978), many employees know what they are to do, but not why they are doing it or how the patterned activities in which they are involved accomplish a given objective. People seek clarification about the organisation's general goals and specific objectives, and the organisation's strategies and achievements. Likewise, management does not always know what employees are doing, or how what they are doing contributes to the organisation's overall objectives. Upward communication is perhaps more important in organisations in the health sector than in many other sectors. The objective of these organisations is to promote the health of individuals and communities. They have to advocate change in order to create supportive environments, they have to put health on the (local and national) political agenda, and they have a duty in campaigning to improve the health of the population they serve. In order to achieve this objective, the management needs a sophisticated understanding of, for example, the environmental conditions influencing health, the needs of their target population, their way of thinking, and their reactions to health campaigns. Much of this information enters the organisation through field level staff members, who are in direct contact with these target populations. If this information fails to reach the management rapidly and accurately, it is almost impossible to make effective management decisions. Therefore, regular meetings at all levels, downward, horizontal and upward, are important for organisations to survive in the environment in which they operate, but also to create mutual understanding within organisations and to obtain a certain level of flexibility in dealing with new challenges. Organisations, as well as people, learn and change through a process of diffusion of ideas and practices.

10.4 Flexibility

Communication and motivation are important factors for the creation of flexibility within organisations. Organisations are often bureaucratic, that is, they tend to standardise workflow. Bureaucratic organisations have great difficulty in adapting to changing circumstances. According to Weick (1979), flexibility is required so that current practices can be modified in the interests of adapting to changes in the environment. Indeed, most organisations will probably have to reach different goals, new target groups, and deal with different (health-related) issues in the future and, indeed, flexibility is a necessity if one wishes to remain ahead of developments in the field. Flexibility requires a continuous programme of organisational development, as well as a policy that creates opportunities for the personal development of staff, and rewards for those who use these opportunities effectively. According to Thompson and Winner (1999:149), flexible organisations are characterised by a constant, open flow of information, and an inbuilt cadre of volunteers or staff members who are both willing and able to respond to changes in the environment. There are limitations to flexibility however. This is expressed nicely by Weick (1979:215) who states: 'the trouble with total flexibility is the organisation cannot over time retain a sense of identity and continuity. Any social unit is defined in part by its history, by what it has done and by what it has chosen repeatedly. Chronic flexibility destroys identity'. We would advise organisations to develop a culture of learning in which all volunteer and staff members contribute to a process of discovering how the organisation can adjust itself to a changing environment with new opportunities. In order to address the complexity of the field of health, and the changes in the environment of organisations, the importance of internally and externally directed communication processes should not be underestimated.

10.5 Leadership

The leadership of an organisation will try to ensure that its staff members contribute to the achievement of organisational goals as much as possible. To this end, employees receive job descriptions indicating clearly what each employee should or should not do. Managers take decisions by processing information with reference to a set of predetermined rules. The manager decides what has to be done and in what way. Organisations using this directive style have the tendency to become bureaucratic and inflexible. All the work processes become standardised. Deviations are discouraged. In terms of communication processes, there is a lot of downward communication and an absence of upward and horizontal communication. Bureaucratic organisations have great difficulty in adapting to changes in their environment. Changes in the environment often lead to internal conflicts and malfunctioning of the organisation as a whole (Mintzberg, 1983). At the other extreme, employees can be given extensive freedom in deciding what should be done, provided that these decisions are discussed at meetings in which staff try to clarify with management what the best decisions are in different situations. This leadership style is termed the participatory style. Clearly, there are many alternatives lying between these two extremes. In the context of the philosophy of health promotion however, the more participatory style is, in our opinion, the more appropriate. Good leaders are inspirational, good listeners, have the capability of reflection, and are able to get the best out of people.

It should be noted that the leadership structure of an organisation may support change in response to changing external and internal conditions, and this is likely to have an effect on individuals within the organisation (Thompson & Kinne, 1999). Organisations will try to attract staff who are willing and able to contribute as much as possible to fulfilling organisational goals. Individual staff members will accept positions within the organisation because they expect to achieve a large proportion of their own goals in this way. Both sets of goals are seldom in complete agreement. Even if they were when the staff member joined the organisation, they may diverge afterwards as the goals of both the individual and the organisation change.

We have stressed the importance of good communication within an organisation to help it to achieve its goals. Motivation of staff is important for the same reason. The effectiveness of the work of any organisation largely depends on the abilities, qualities and motivation of the staff. In terms of motivation, staff members need to know clearly what their task is, they must consider the task to be important and realistic, both for themselves and in relation to the mission or aim to which the task is contributing. Staff members are more likely to consider the task to be important if the information they have provided is used in decision making with regard to the direction of activities and programmes. Hence, it is desirable for organisations to discuss this direction openly with staff members at all levels. Moreover, the time people are allowed to spend on certain tasks contains motivational aspects. Generally, people tend to lose motivation if they are unable to complete a task. Motivation of staff is also influenced by the organisation's reward system. Consider our discussion in section 3.2 about learning. Rewards can be material and financial, but also social. Receiving support from management, superiors and peers is an important motivational force.

10.6 The organisation of intersectoral collaboration

Health promotion does not belong to any specific organisation or to any specific place inside an organisation. It takes the form of inter-organisational programmes. This means that some type of 'new organisation' has to be developed, one that exists separately from the contributing organisations. Many collaborative health promotion activities rely on partnerships between organisations, either between private organisations, governmental and non-governmental organisations, or between community and voluntary organisations; but developing partnerships with different organisations and people is no easy task, especially when organisations are going to work together for the first time. Generally speaking, most health promotion activities start as a temporary organisation, such as a project. However, in health promotion the aim is to become sustainable. Growing from a specific project towards sustainability requires structured inputs and good project management. It is not possible to give a clear blueprint of potentially sustainable projects for the organisation. An interesting approach to this is what is called 'goal directed project management', as developed by Andersen *et al.* (1995). This approach has been developed within the field of computer technology, but also applies well to the field of health education and promotion. Central to their approach is the PSO concept. PSO stands for People, System and Organisation. PSO projects are those where the development of a system (for example, a physical product, an intervention or a specific health service) and development of people and organisations occur simultaneously. The authors define a project as: a unique task, which is designed to attain specific results, which requires a variety of resources, and which is limited in time (Andersen *et al.*, 1995:24). Although this definition is restrictive in that it refers to a unique, non-recurring task that is limited in time, the idea of a project organisation can be very helpful in developing sustainable programmes. A good example can be found in a study conducted by Withag (1990) who applied the project organisation concept in order to develop a sustainable health-promoting workplace in a middle range production organisation.

10.6.1 Characteristics of a project organisation

Projects have some characteristic features that give rise to certain leadership and management problems. A project involves new and unknown tasks, leads to changes in people's daily work and living conditions, requires the right people at the right time, and is subject to strict deadlines.

Required tasks
At the onset of any project, the activities that need to be performed are unknown in detail and, consequently, there is no detailed blueprint for how to proceed in order to achieve the desired results. For people, getting involved in a community-based health promotion project may be quite unfamiliar, involving working in a different area or setting, and working with new people. For example, an epidemiologist employed by a municipal health service may be a specialist in survey research but have no experience in the organisation of group discussions about health issues. Hence, the tasks required are new. Moreover, the people involved have different backgrounds and usually are not used to working together in the composition of the project.

When projects are being organised, both the principles governing relationships between parties involved and the practical consequences of these relationships must be defined, as well as the roles and responsibilities each of the participants is both *willing* and *able* to take on. It is important to realise that a project in fact is a change process that changes people's working environment, as well as their understanding of the organisation of which they are part and the other organisations with which they work. The work of developing relationships between the participants and attitudes towards the tasks is an essential part of the project. Hence, the process-oriented elements are very important. Consequently, project management equals change management.

The attainment of results
A project is established to achieve a specific result, such as an effective intervention, a sound action plan, or a programme that has to prove itself to become sustainable. An important issue in relation to this is agreement about the aims and objectives. In health promotion projects, the overall aim is usually defined beforehand, and projects are organised around this aim (see section 7.7). Specific aims, however, usually develop throughout the process as a result of cooperation. Andersen *et al.* (1995) differentiate the extent to which the people who benefit from the results of a project have the opportunity to participate in the project. At one extreme, they position the purely specialist projects, in which all the work is performed by experts, without any form of cooperation or consultation with those for whom the project has been developed. Such projects can be characterised as a direct contact change situation as described in section 7.5, and do not exceed level 2 on the ladder of participation, that is, participation by information (see Table 7.1). Traditional health education projects often appear in this form. In these projects, aims and objectives are typically formulated beforehand. At the other extreme, we can position the purely process-oriented projects, where little or no consideration is given to planning the technical outcome (i.e. an intervention). Everyone is encouraged to become involved, and the project is allowed to be dominated by whatever problems and possibilities the participants see as being most important at any given time. The process itself (the interaction between people and what it leads to) determines the progress of the project. This type of project resembles the immanent change project and reflects the highest level of participation.

Variety of resources

For effective partnerships it is necessary that all those concerned allocate sufficient resources for a project from the very outset. Andersen *et al.* (1995) mention various reasons why organisations are reluctant to commit resources to projects. Similar problems have been reported in literature on health promotion projects (*cf.* Koelen, 2000; Boonekamp *et al.*, 1995; Graham & Bois, 1997). We summarise them in Table 10.1.

Table 10.1 Why organisations are reluctant to commit resources.

- They hope that staff can participate on top of their regular job; without reduction of original responsibilities
- They do not understand why the project should take such long time
- They do not understand that a reduction in resources means a reduction in quality
- They do not accept the time and effort required in process oriented projects, due to their experience with technical work
- There is a limited understanding of what it takes to achieve good results in preocess oriented projects
- Practical problems to release the required people at the required time
- Projects bring together people with different expertise, who are not used to work togetherw

Time constraints

Especially when projects are to be financed by external agencies, there is a fixed deadline for obtaining funding, and this might hamper the involvement of important stakeholders, and in particular members of the target population (*cf.* Graham & Bois, 1997; Wagemakers, 2000; Koelen *et al.*, 2001). Equally, external deadlines are set for the completion date. Usually in such situations the focus is on this deadline instead of on the process of developing the content around which the project was built. Even though it may be difficult, in order to prevent a project from failing to reach its goals, it is important to set out a time plan with milestones. A milestone describes *what* the project should achieve by a certain moment (not how) and shows the dependencies between them. Milestones help to ensure that the project is on the right track. It should be noted, however, that flexibility remains important. Sometimes achievements take longer than expected, due for example, to unforeseen circumstances, or just because steps take more time than could have been predicted. On the other hand however, sometimes in certain stages a project can gain time by hiring experts either to solve a problem or to advise on how to approach that problem.

10.7 Factors influencing the success and sustainability of collective action

Most health promotion programmes begin as a project, but projects have specific aims, defined budgets and defined time limits. With health promotion programmes, we try to achieve lasting, healthy living patterns and conditions. However, achieving behavioural change at the individual level requires long-term attention to an issue. Consequently, programmes should also be enduring. By working through participatory methods, health promotion programmes are expected to become sustainable, that is, they maintain services without extra external input. This means that the networks and activities initiated in the project have to become permanently woven into the local structures. In the process of active participation, community members and organisations work together to build the new reality, and the resulting structure is 'their own'. As Green and Kreuter (1991:46) state: 'programmes conceived and developed apart from the spirit and the day-to-day workings of a community are, by definition, outside that community. In such cases, when the initial resources dry up or the intervention period comes to an end, the programme is not only over, it is gone!' Genuine participation and commitment are essential in order to make programmes real parts of the community, to generate a sense of ownership, and to achieve sustainability,

Based on our experiences in community development and in community-based health promotion (Koelen, 2000; Koelen & Vaandrager, 1997; Boonekamp *et al.*, 1995) and based on the experiences of others as found in literature, we can identify seven factors that are important in achieving and sustaining intersectoral or collaborative action. These are: communication and information, common aims and objectives, visibility, management, community participation, political involvement and policy development.

Communication and information

One important part of networking is to create communication structures in order to share ideas, experience and information. Health promotion is not a one-way information providing activity; it involves an interactive exchange of information between all the parties involved. Organisations and people learn and change through a process of diffusion of ideas and practices. Networks in the community facilitate such diffusion. Therefore, information and communication need attention. This issue is important on both an organisational and an individual level. On the organisational level, health promotion is an ongoing process of decision making that requires a flow of regular inputs of information from and about the community and between all the people involved. It requires a regular assessment of needs, discussion with community members, and open channels to receive signals from the community. On the individual level, it is important to place emphasis on building people's capacities to access external information when they need it, on developing their ability to experiment and draw conclusions, and on their individual and collective ability to take sound decisions. This means that it is necessary to actively facilitate the communication process and to put emphasis on (citizen) self-activity. Consultation media (telephone, database, Teletext or Internet) are suitable for supplying people with information at times when they are actively searching for this information.

Common aims and objectives

Stakeholders need to recognise common ground and responsibilities, and they have to agree on a common goal for the issue on which they are working. It is also necessary to 'agree to disagree' on all the other things (Milio, 1997). This is, for example, an important precondition for working with the commercial sector or for cooperation between organisations with clear differences in mission. In addition, a clear structure and allocation of tasks is required. The multi-disciplinary nature of networks involves a variety of skills and expertise, and therefore insight into the possibilities and expectations of all actors involved. Successful collaboration requires clear role definitions of participants, based on their own possibilities and wishes. A clear structure, outlining the goals of each activity, roles, responsibilities, and a timetable for activities helps to structure the process. It is also necessary that the outline has some flexibility, in order to respond to changes and to incorporate learning experiences into programme planning.

Visibility

Visibility is important for collaboration and participation. It functions as an incentive for involvement, action and continuation. Visibility firstly refers to *visibility of activities*. This is important not only for the community at large, but also for the participants in action. Visibility can be achieved by being present on a stand at community events, but also through specific materials, media attention, and local reports. Visibility also refers to *visibility of outcomes*. This requires the regular evaluation of activities during several phases of the programme, and the active feedback of results to the project team. The idea that, by working together, things can be achieved that each participant on his or her own could not achieve (the principle of synergy) is particularly important. Visible outcomes function not only as an incentive for all participants in the process, but also as a means of getting political and financial support from decision makers. Finally, *visibility of the individual contributions* is productive. It must be clear what the participants themselves are contributing. People need to see or feel that they are important to the progress of the project.

Management

The management process of intersectoral collaboration needs to receive specific attention. The main problem may not be identifying 'what to do' but finding out 'how to get it done'. Participatory processes require certain leadership and a supporting framework. The manager or system integrator (*cf.* Koelen & Brouwers, 1990) fulfils an important role. Such a manager needs to be:
- acceptable to the partners
- flexible and reliable
- practical, using available resources
- good at following up on decisions
- enthusiastic and motivated, also a good motivator
- visionary and a good listener
- committed to the programme, and have enough time available.

The manager has to maintain a good network communication infrastructure and encourage the sharing of ideas, experience and information. Management includes initiating debates and making

Chapter 10

realistic plans that reflect the wishes and possibilities of those involved in the programme. Good communication structures, clear aims and objectives, and the well-defined roles and responsibilities of participants help to structure the process.

Community participation
Community participation is such an important part of collaborative action that we need to discuss it separately. As we argued in section 7.7.1, simply approaching community members and asking them to participate in project planning and implementation is inappropriate and will not be successful. To achieve a satisfactory level of community involvement, the following points at least need to be addressed:
- activities have to be consistent with community needs
- members must be involved in decision making and must have their own, clear responsibilities
- the importance of their contribution and the benefits to members themselves must be clear
- contributions from volunteers must be visible
- rapid implementation of activities, once developed, is an essential factor in sustaining community involvement.

Furthermore, involvement of community members in research and interpretation of research results is an important stimulating factor for sustaining community participation. In the European Super project, a community-based nutrition promotion programme (*cf.* Koelen, 2000; Vaandrager, 1995), we found that asking community members to comment on the research results of process-and-effect evaluations through group discussion was helpful in understanding the reasons for 'successes and failures', therefore enabling the improvement of certain aspects of the programme. In addition, it made clear to community members that their opinions were being taken seriously.

Political involvement
The political environment is of major importance for health organisations and their activities. Politicians and decision makers influence a range of activities and possibilities, either at national or local level. The actual impact of politics and decision makers depends heavily on the national and local political situation, and therefore political commitment takes different forms. Political support is necessary for important reasons. Firstly, given that the (local)

government is responsible for health, political commitment is a basic necessity for the development and implementation of reform strategies. Having commitment and formal agreement at the political level and the level of decision makers is facilitative in many ways (see section 7.7). The credibility of organisations and their projects is enhanced and their profiles rise. Developing collaborations becomes easier, and financial and other relevant resources can be secured. In the end, a formal political agreement helps to improve sustainability.

Policy development

Policy development is an essential condition for sustainability. It can help to convince key decision makers on a higher level, such as directors of local organisations, supermarket chains and local politicians. Policy development is necessary to institutionalise health promotion programmes. Thinking about policy development should be included right from the beginning rather than when the project is nearing its end. However, it is hard to convince key decision makers without having any concrete evidence. Involvement of decision makers and politicians is essential for policy development, as are the visibility of actions, visibility of results, and visibility of participants in the project.

10.8 Chapter summary

In this chapter we have discussed the functioning of organisations within a changing environment. Based on the open systems theory, we pointed out the necessity for organisations to adapt to these changing environments. We argued that clear and flexible leadership, as well as clear and flexible internal communication structures, are essential for the survival of organisations, both with a view to organisations' flexibility, and with a view to the motivation of staff members. With regard to external communication we identified two trajectories: the external-internal trajectory (communication with conditional and other input relation groups), and the internal-external trajectory (communication with output groups, groups serving related objectives, and normative relation groups). Special attention was given to the organisation of intersectoral collaboration, and factors influencing the success and sustainability of collective action.

11. Health promotion ethics

Health education and health promotion professionals are engaged in activities that explicitly aim to enable individuals, organisations and communities to achieve their potential to enhance their own lives and the lives of other people. As we have seen throughout this book, within this scope a range of interventions can be used. In many instances these interventions touch upon dearly prized values and raise important ethical concerns (Yeo, 1993). The ability and possibility for health professionals to influence people and communities are increasing, both as a result of developments in communication and information technology, and as a result of advances in science, medicine and engineering. This ability can be used not only in the interests of humanity, but also to cause serious harm, a development that implies that health educators and health promoters must take added responsibility for their actions. We see similar developments in other fields. Current military technology, for example, is much more capable of damaging humanity than the bow and arrow.

Health promotion is interdisciplinary and inter-professional. Many organisations, departments, institutions and individuals from a variety of disciplines are involved. Each discipline has not only its own specific domain of knowledge and information, but also its own origin, objectives, standards, and interests. The behaviour of professionals is influenced by the organisation that employs them, the people with and for whom they work, their colleagues, the professional values in which they have been trained and by the wider society to which they belong. This is illustrated in Figure 11.1, the square of loyalties (Proost, 1993). Each of these groups of people has ideas about how health professionals should behave, but these ideas may conflict with each other to some extent. The group to which one is most inclined to listen will depend partly on the values of this group and partly on the power that different groups may have over the health professional.

In this chapter we discuss several decisions a health professional needs to make, and raise some ethical questions for which health workers, and the organisations they represent, should find answers that satisfy

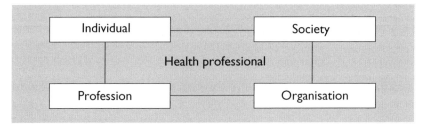

Figure 11.1 A health worker's square of loyalties.

their consciences. It is not our intention to say how one should deal with these issues; that is a task for the reader.

11.1 Culture, norms and values

Interventions in health education often aim to persuade or assist individuals in modifying behaviour in a way conducive to their health. One strives to help people to form more considered opinions about their situation and to take more rational decisions, making optimal use of scientific research findings. In the past it was assumed that the application of science automatically led to an improvement in our lives. The modern association between science and warfare has caused many people to reassess this view. Some now believe that non-scientific solutions to problems are almost always better. We do not share this extreme view. We believe that science has been used more often to improve society than to bring about undesirable changes, although we accept that the latter also occur. For example, the development and application of DDT provided a valuable tool for controlling malaria. Unfortunately, it also led to the deposition of harmful residues in mothers' milk.

Continued economic growth and higher per capita incomes have been the goals of most industrial societies for many years. Diminishing natural resources and increasing problems with pollution and environmental damage have stimulated many societies to reassess these goals. The catch is that many members of these societies want the advantages of economic growth without accepting or having regard for the disadvantages. Pressure groups may fight for higher incomes for their members but show little concern for the environmental impact of increased production and consumption.

The decision about whether or not to stimulate further economic growth will depend partly on the present standard of living enjoyed by the majority of members of any given society. Those living in industrially advanced countries will probably answer this question in a different way from those living in poorer countries. Some people from industrialised countries who work in less industrialised countries assume that changes they would consider desirable in their home society should also be considered desirable in their host country. However, even apparently fundamental questions relating to the improvement of health and prolongation of life may be answered in different ways by different societies. Consider the differences in national policies on euthanasia and abortion in European countries, and the differences in public opinion about these issues within these countries. Opinions about desirable changes are influenced strongly by personal views about what constitutes a good society. These views are the result of extended cultural development processes and of personal experiences.

Population control and family planning have become important issues in many countries, especially in densely populated areas such as Java and Bangladesh. However, we find there are many clashes between various sets of beliefs, norms and values, which make the implementation of population control extremely difficult. On the one hand, a government may decide to promote family planning in rural areas because the country cannot support more people from its agricultural resources. On the other hand, the norms and religious values of the people favour large families. Furthermore, some cultures place special value on having many children because of their importance as a labour resource and as a form of insurance for the parents in their old age. Government programmes to promote family planning then lead to serious clashes in personal values, as we saw in India during the 1970s. Health professionals in these situations face some extremely difficult decisions about how to match their own values with those of the community they work for and with.

11.2 Responsibility

Health education and health promotion is regarded as a skilled activity that is usually undertaken by professionals. Most health professionals and other workers in this field have had more formal education than the average population. This poses problems of power, responsibilities and knowledge. Yet, as Pattison and Player (1990:65) argue, to what extent do they have the right to change others? Do they really know best? Do other members of society not have a right to have their perceptions of health and illness taken seriously, rather than having their knowledge and beliefs dismissed as 'folk tales'? In addition, health workers emphasise the importance of good health, whereas others may consider other goals to be more important than being healthy.

A major aim of health education and health promotion is to enhance personal autonomy by increasing the individual's freedom to make his or her own decisions. This is what is meant by the concepts of enabling and empowerment. Similarly, health promotion strives towards the empowerment of communities and their ownership and control of their own endeavours and destinies. However, enabling is not a matter of saying 'You are responsible', as in laying the blame or burden on someone. Nor is it a matter of treating people as victims who can be helped only by the grace of some benign intervener (Yeo, 1993:233). At times we forget that increased freedom also brings with it more responsibilities for the consequences our actions may have for our fellow man.

Improving their health is an important goal for most people, but it is not their only goal in life, and it may be in conflict with other goals. A person may also enjoy an exuberant life style, going to parties with nice food and drink. He or she may realise that this life style increases the chance of dying early but be convinced that it is better to have a short, pleasant life than a long, but dull one. Should the health professional try to convince this person to change to a healthy life style? The authors of this book do not see it as their task to answer this question for you, the reader, but you cannot avoid trying to find an answer for this question for yourself. One consideration could be that one's choice of lifestyle has consequences not just for oneself but also for other persons in one's environment - for instance, children. Another consideration could be that health professionals will probably get more recognition among colleagues if they opt to promote a healthy way of life than if they allow complete autonomy to clients to make their own decision (see Figure 11.1). To us, there is no doubt that enhancing the autonomy of the clients requires helping them to obtain the best possible knowledge on the consequences of the choices they make. However, their choice will be based not only on knowledge but also on values. On whose values?

11.3 Nature of interventions

The work of the health educator is bound to involve some intervention in the lives of other people. A whole range of interventions is possible and, in order to decide what is the best practice, the health worker has to consider several questions, such as:
- Which problems will we alert people to?
- Which problems, raised by people, do we pay attention to?
- Should we create anxiety? If yes, how much, and does it serve a useful purpose?
- What do we do when the results of a change are only partially known?
- Which criteria do we use to evaluate alternatives?

Generally, the sooner people are aware of a problem the greater the chance of finding a solution to it. For example, cancer is much easier to cure in its early stages than when it has already caused substantial damage. HIV/AIDS is much easier to prevent than to cure. Health professionals favouring a participatory approach often start with the felt needs of the people or the community and not with what professionals consider to be their needs. A result of this approach may be that one takes too much time to find a good solution for the health problem. People generally appear to change their behaviour faster when they are slightly, but not very, anxious, and are presented with a practical way of reducing this anxiety (see Chapter 3). However, health professionals have an extremely difficult task when they recognise that an individual has a problem for which no solution is known, as is the case with some diseases.

Interventions can take many different forms. To mention just a few (based on the work of Seedhouse, 1992):

- Interventions that are requested and agreed. For example, the intervention that takes place when a person consults a dietician voluntarily.
- Interventions that are not requested, but which the 'target' finds desirable. For example, the intervention that takes place when a health visitor or district nurse calls unannounced and finds an old lady alone without heating, and too proud to ask for help.
- Interventions not requested and probably not desired by (parts of) the community. Many mass media campaigns take this form. For example, a campaign addressing the consequences of alcohol consumption or a campaign explaining why one should stop smoking.
- Interventions that are enforced by law. For example, a prohibition on the sale of alcoholic drinks in sports canteens or the introduction of smoke-free public buildings.

It is clear that each of these will need different consideration. It becomes even more complicated if we consider that, quite often, alternative courses of action addressed in intervention programmes are only partly known. Should the health professionals explain these uncertainties? What should they do when asked for concrete advice? When they explain the uncertainties, is it because it is in the person's best interests to understand them, or is it because the person might hold the health professional responsible if results were not as had been expected? In other words, are the professionals merely protecting themselves against criticism? More and more people sue professionals for unanticipated and undesired effects of their recommendations.

Interventions discussed so far are based on the individual behaviour and lifestyle approach. Health promotion starts from the notion that both individual *and* structural elements have to be addressed. Therefore it is also important to consider the systems approach, in which interventions focus on the *system* that impinges on health, or, in the words of Green and Reaburn (1988:153), on the social, economic, political, institutional, cultural, legislative, industrial and physical environment in which behaviour takes place. Changes in the environment can be conducive to health, as is expressed in the phrase 'make healthy choices easy choices', but can also involve individual, social or economic restrictions. According to Yeo (1993), the individual approach is aligned with interventions towards the voluntary end of the intervention continuum, whereas the systems approach is aligned with interventions towards the non-voluntary or even coercive end of the continuum. For example, a law regulating driving while under the influence of alcohol may remarkably reduce the number of accidents, but it also restricts individual freedom of choice, which is considered an important human right. Also, systems interventions to, for example, re-orient health services may require considerable financial resources, which, in the end, have to come from tax payers or the consumers.

11.4 Relationships

In all ethical considerations, relationships are crucial and, at the same time, lead to important questions. Northouse & Northouse (1992), for example, consider four dimensions to be important in the relationship between health care professionals and their clients.

- Health workers should help people to make decisions that are beneficial to them. But on the basis of which values do they decide what is beneficial?
- They should not be paternalistic; that is, they should only provide help that people want. But what should they do if people are not aware that their present way of life may cause serious health problems for them at some time in the future?
- They should promote people's autonomy to enable them to decide for themselves how to live their lives. But what should health workers do when asked to make a difficult decision *for* them?
- Health workers should be honest, but what happens if they are? The truth about any situation is rarely clear and seldom simple. For example, it may be desirable that people stop eating certain kinds of foods for the good of their cardiovascular system, whereas at the same time it may be true that social class position, poor living conditions and stress also contribute to heart disease (Pattison & Player, 1990). Presentation of all facts is incompatible with the notion of getting a clear message across, whereas the latter is incompatible with telling the truth.

Health educators and health promoters should certainly consider these dimensions when deciding on their relationships with people, but difficult ethical decisions are involved in applying them. They may conflict with one another, and this could have undesirable consequences for the individual, or for the individual's trust in the professional.

11.5 Codes of ethics

It is not easy to give clear and enduring guidelines that will direct ethical decision making. Yet, some basic ethical considerations should be at the heart of any health-promoting intervention. According to the humanistic view of the WHO, a strong ethical framework includes respect for individual choice, personal autonomy and the avoidance of harm, and applies to both individual and social aspects of health care and research. In the *Health for All in the 21st Century* (WHO, 1998:21) document it is stated that 'ethics will guide all aspects of Health for All planning and implementation'. A distinction is made between (a) the conduct of health professionals, (b) policies and priorities for health systems and health services, and (c) science, research and technology (see Table 3.1).

In August 2000, the *Journal of Health Education* published a code of ethics for the health education profession. The preamble is that: 'The health education profession is dedicated to excellence in the practice of promoting individual, family, organisational, and community health. Guided by common ideals, health educators are responsible for upholding integrity and ethics of the profession as they face the daily challenges of making decisions. By acknowledging the value of diversity in society and embracing a cross-cultural approach, health educators support the worth, dignity, potential, and uniqueness of all people.'

The code of ethics is grounded in fundamental ethical principles that underlie all health care services and covers the key issues as mentioned by WHO (see Table 11.1): respect for autonomy, promotion of social justice, active promotion of good, and avoidance of harm. The code consists of six articles, which we briefly summarise below. For the complete text, refer to the *Journal of Health Education* (2000, 31:216-218). In the articles it is mentioned that health educators have:
1. *Responsibility to the public*, this refers to the ultimate responsibility of health educators to educate people for the purpose of promoting, maintaining, and improving individual, family, and community

Table 11.1 Ethics (WHO, 1998).

Ethics will guide all aspects of Health for All planning and implementation	
The conduct of health professionals	• Promote health and prevent and treat disease
	• Provide compassionate care across the life span
	• Respect individual choice, confidentiality and autonomy
	• Avoid harm
	• Appreciate diverse values and needs
Policies and priorities for health systems and services	• Work for equity and social justice in access to health care
	• Involve patients and other members of the public in setting priorities for access to health interventions
	• Incorporate equity considerations into decision-making about resource allocation within and between countries
	• Educate health workers and the public about ethical principles
Science, research and technology	• Monitor and update, as necessary, ethical norms for research
	• Anticipate ethical implications of advances in science, and technology for health
	• Apply internationally codes of ethics
	• Ensure that agreed ethical standards guide future work on the human genome
	• Ensure that quality in health systems and services is assessed and promoted

health. In case of conflicting issues, '.. health educators must consider all issues and give priority to those that promote wellness and quality of living through principles of self-determination and freedom of choice for the individual.'

2. *Responsibility to the profession*, stating, 'health educators are responsible for their professional behaviour, for the reputation of their profession, and for promoting ethical conduct among their colleagues.'

3. *Responsibility to employers*: 'health educators recognise the boundaries of their professional competence and are accountable for their professional activities and actions.'

4. *Responsibility in the delivery of health education*: 'health educators promote integrity in the delivery of health education. They respect the rights, dignity, confidentiality, and worth of all people by

adapting strategies and methods to meet the needs of diverse populations and communities.'

5. *Responsibility in research and evaluation*: 'health educators contribute to the health of the population and to the profession through research and evaluation activities. When planning and conducting research or evaluation, health educators do so in accordance with federal and state laws and regulations, organisational and institutional policies, and professional standards.'

6. *Responsibility in professional preparation*: 'Those involved in the preparation and training of health educators have an obligation to accord learners the same respect and treatment given other groups by providing quality education that benefits the profession and the public.'

The issues addressed in this chapter are only a few out of a wide range of ethical concerns with which health workers are faced. Since society, science, health-related topics and so forth are liable to continuous changes, ethical concerns also change continuously. We suggest it is important to think about ethical issues again and again, but also to consider the ethics relating to each intervention on its own, in the context in which it is implemented. The presented code of ethics may serve as a guideline.

11.6 Chapter summary

By the very nature of their work, health professionals intervene in the lives of individuals, organisations and communities. Consequently, they may face difficult ethical choices. In this chapter several ethical issues and questions have been addressed, relating to culture, values and norms; responsibilities; the nature of interventions; and relationships. Existing 'codes of ethics' have been presented; these may help health professionals to find their own way. We are not in a position to give solutions or clear answers for every situation in which health professionals are involved, but we stress the importance of thinking about ethical issues again and again, relating to each intervention, in the context in which it is implemented.

Glossary

Absolute standards: Standards used in the formulation of objectives for health promotion programmes, where expectations are of 100 per cent success.

Acceptance (private conformity): Conformity to group norms because people are persuaded and truly believe the group is right; they accept and internalise the group norms as their own beliefs.

Action research: Research aiming to analyse a specific situation. Research results are immediately fed back into a programme for decision making in that situation.

Action stage: The stage in which individuals make specific modifications in their lifestyle (Transtheoretical model of behaviour change).

Adopter categories: Members of a social unit, classified on the basis of speed of adoption of innovations of a certain type, e.g. innovations based on health research.

Adoption (of innovation): Decision to apply an innovation and to continue to use it.

Adoption process (with regard to an innovation): The change process that takes place on an individual level between initial awareness of the innovation and the final decision to use it.

Attitude: A relatively enduring tendency to respond to an object in a way that reflects a positive or negative evaluation of that object. An attitude object can be another person, a thing, or a specific behaviour.

Attribution to stable causes: Ascribing (attributing) the cause of a certain consequence to a factor which is relatively difficult to change over time (e.g. ability; task difficulty).

Attribution to unstable causes: Ascribing (attributing) the cause of a certain consequence to a factor which is relatively easy to change over time (e.g. effort; luck).

Awareness raising: Becoming aware of causes and consequences of certain problem behaviour by means of experiences, observations and confrontations. Similar to *Consciousness raising*.

Behavioural beliefs: Beliefs about the consequences of performing behaviour.

Behavioural diagnosis: A systematic analysis of health-related behaviour.

Behavioural objectives: Description of behaviour to be addressed in health interventions.

Biomedical research approach: Research to discover, predict and control certain phenomena. Results from this type of research are used to find support for a hypothesis, or to show whether or not an intervention is effective. The researcher acts as an external observer. See *Traditional research approach.*

Bureaucratic organisation: Organisation characterised by central leadership, hierarchical regulation of functionaries, rigid decision processes according to general rules and routine procedures.

Change agent: Person who tries to stimulate change among people or organisations. A health promotion professional is an example of a change agent.

Cognitive map: Codes and symbols of transitory experiences retained in symbols for memory representation.

Cohesion: Those aspects binding groups or societies together, such as feelings of belonging to a group or a community, and feelings of inter-relatedness.

Communication: Transactional process of sending and receiving messages through channels, which establishes common meanings between a source and a receiver.

Communication channel: The textual, auditive, or visual way in which a message is transferred.

Communication process: Process that takes place when people or groups communicate with each other.

Community: Groups of people who identify themselves by their group membership, sharing a common interest, common social institutions and common social control components.

Community action for health: Collective efforts directed towards increasing community control over determinants of health, and thereby improving health.

Community coalitions: Formal or informal alliances of individuals, representing diverse organisations, interest groups, actions or constituencies, which combine their human and material resources.

Community participation: A process whereby community members take part in identification of their needs, priority setting, identifying and obtaining means, including the development, implementation and evaluation of those means in terms of outcomes.

Compatibility: The degree to which an innovation is consistent with socio-cultural values, beliefs, needs or experiences of a group.

Complexity: The degree to which an innovation is perceived as difficult to understand or difficult to use.

Compliance (public conformity): Conformity to group norms, restricted to a specific situation in which the norm is important.

Conformity: The convergence of an individual's thoughts, feelings and behaviour toward a group norm.

Consciousness raising: Becoming aware of causes and consequences of problem behaviour, for example by means of experiences, observations and confrontations. Similar to *Awareness raising*.

Contemplation stage: The stage in which individuals are aware that a (health) problem exists and of the need for behaviour change (Transtheoretical model of behaviour change).

Control group: Group in experimental research *not* exposed to a treatment, e.g. to a new drug. See *Experimental group*.

Coping appraisal: Assessment of the perceived effectiveness of recommended behaviour.

Counselling model of dialogue: Client-centred dialogue that helps people to make decisions by clarifying their feelings and experiences in order to create an encouraging atmosphere.

Cue to action: Some form of awareness of a threat that makes a person feel the need to take action.

Culture: All norms, values, knowledge, ideas, art, science, laws, habits, and institutions of a social system, e.g. a community.

Decision making: All considerations that play a role in making a choice.

Decoding: The process by which a receiver transforms signals in messages into cognitions. See *Encoding*.

Dependent variable: That aspect of a person's behaviour (e.g. smoking behaviour) that is measured after the manipulation of the independent variable (e.g. an anti-smoking campaign). See *Independent variable*.

Diagnosis-prescription model of dialogue: A typical, expert-led dialogue, where the expert asks a series of questions, diagnoses the nature of the problem and its possible causes, and gives prescriptions and advice. Clients merely have a passive role.

Dialogue: A one-to-one communication also referred to as mutual discussion, counselling, or personal instruction.

Diffusion research: Research into the way in which innovations are generally spread among the members of a social system. See also *Adoption research,* with which it is usually combined.

Diffusion: The process by which an innovation is communicated through certain channels over time among members of a social system.

Disease prevention: Collective measurers to prevent specific diseases, e.g. vaccination or screening programmes.

Documentary-historical inquiry: Research analysing artefacts, such as archives literature, medical records, or minutes.

Educational communication: Communication to help individuals identify their needs, to improve their problem solving capacities, to gain skills, and improve self-confidence.

Effectiveness evaluation: Evaluation of the extent to which an intervention programme has achieved its intervention objectives.

Efficacy expectation: The conviction that one can execute the behaviour required to produce desired outcomes.

Efficiency evaluation: Evaluation of the (cost-) effectiveness of an intervention programme. It gives insight into the achieved goals in comparison with alternative or competing interventions.

Empowerment: The process through which individuals gain greater control over decisions and actions affecting their life, including their health.

Enabling factors: Factors that facilitate individuals or groups to perform an action, e.g. skills.

Encoding: Cognitive process of transforming ideas and feelings into symbols, and subsequently organising them into a message. See *Decoding*.

Endogenous determinants of health: Determinants that affect health from the inside, i.e. biological factors, which may be hereditary or acquired in the course of life.

Entertainment-education: The process of designing and implementing a media message both to entertain and educate, in order to increase audience members' knowledge about an educational issue, create favourable attitudes, and change overt behaviour.

Environmental diagnosis: Analysis of factors in the physical and social environment that can be causally linked to (health-related) behaviour.

Environmental objectives: Describe the conditions in the environment necessary to facilitate or support behavioural change.

Evaluation (1): A review of results that are achieved in relation to the aims and objectives of a programme.

Evaluation (2): A policy management instrument to collect and analyse information in a systematically and objectively manner. The relevance, effect and consequences of activities are determined in order to improve present and future activities in line with policy.

Exogenous determinants of health: External influences on health, relating to physical environment, lifestyle factors and social environment.

Experimental group: The group in experimental research that is exposed to a treatment, e.g. to a new drug. See *Control group*.

Experimental research: Research aimed at studying causal relations between two or more variables, in tightly controlled conditions (usually in laboratory settings), using a design with an *experimental group* and a *control group*, both receiving a *pre-test (2nd description)* and a *post-test*.

External attribution: Ascribing (attributing) the cause of a certain consequence to environmental causes, i.e. external to the person. See *Internal attribution*.

External validity: The extent to which observed results of a study can be generalised to other settings and populations with similar characteristics.

Folk media: Communication media that do not use modern technology, but are based on traditional communication methods, such as drama or puppet shows.

Frame of reference: An individual's cognitive representation, on the basis of which he or she judges or acts. The frame is based on pre-existing knowledge and on personal history: culture, norms, and values that have been learned in the social groups to which the individual belongs.

Grassroots coalitions: Coalitions which are organised by volunteers in times of crisis to pressure policy makers to act, such as pressure groups. See *Coalitions*.

Health: A state of complete physical, social and mental well-being, which enables people to lead an individually, socially and economically productive life.

Health care policy: Policy concerned with (the organisation of) diagnostics, treatment, nursing, and health care issues.

Health determinants: Factors that determine the health status of individuals and populations, i.e. endogenous determinants, exogenous determinants, and the system of health care.

Health education: Consciously constructed opportunities for learning, together with (representatives of) the target population, involving some form of communication designed to improve health literacy, including improving knowledge, and developing life skills that are conducive to individual and community health.

Health objectives: Describe health issues to be addressed in health interventions, for whom (targets), which benefit should be achieved, and within what timeframe.

Health promotion: The process of enabling individuals and communities to increase control over, and to improve, their health.

Health protection: Measures to reduce the negative health influences of harmful conditions at home, at work, or in leisure time.

Healthy public policy: Policy in the many and diverse fields which support the promotion of health.

Historical standards: Standards used in formulation of objectives for health promotion programmes, where expectations are derived from the success of previous and comparable programmes.

Hybrid media: The group of media that are based on information and computer technology (ICT).

Independent variable: The condition or stimulus that a researcher manipulates or has under control (e.g. an anti-smoking campaign), and of which the effect is measured on a pre-determined dependent variable (e.g. smoking behaviour). See *Dependent variable*.

Information and computer technology: Electronic systems for storing, retrieving, transmitting, receiving and processing information.

Informational communication: The conscious communication of information to help people to form sound opinions and make good decisions.

Innovation: An idea, practice, or object perceived as new by an individual.

Internal attribution: Ascribing (attributing) the cause of a certain consequence to the person. See *External attribution*.

Internal validity: The extent to which a research design permits causal conclusions to be reached about the effect of the independent variable on the dependent variable. (See *Dependent variable* and *Independent variable*.) Research is internally valid when the causal relation between the independent variable and the dependent variable, as found in the research, is also existent in reality.

Interpersonal communication, non-mediated: Face-to-face interaction between two or more people, in which the parties interact at the same time and in the same place, without a technical device.

Interpersonal communication, mediated: Communication processes where face-to-face communication is mediated by technical devices, for example telephone, electronic mail messages, video conferencing, or letters.

Intersectoral collaboration: A recognised relationship between (parts of) different sectors of society that has been formed to take action on an issue to achieve health outcomes in a way which is more effective, efficient or sustainable than might be achieved by the health sector acting alone.

Intersectoral policy: Policy that lies outside the strict public health sphere but still involves the prevention of damage to health.

Intervention objectives: Description of cognitive and/or psychomotor elements that will be addressed in health interventions.

Latitude of acceptance: The range of positions on a judgement scale that a receiver finds acceptable.

Latitude of non-commitment: The range of positions on a judgement scale that a receiver neither accepts nor rejects.

Latitude of rejection: The range of positions on a judgement scale that a receiver finds unacceptable.

Law of Effect: An action that leads to a desirable outcome is likely to be repeated in similar circumstances.

Leadership: Directing, influencing and controlling of others in pursuit of a group goal.

Learning: Acquiring or improving the ability to perform a behavioural pattern through experience and practice.

Maintenance stage: The stage in which individuals have changed their behaviour and make a great effort to prevent relapse and to consolidate.

Management: The executive function of planning, organising, co-ordinating, directing, controlling and supervising an organisation.

Mass media: Media where the communication process is public, diverse, indirect, via a technical medium, basically one-sided, and usually addressed to a large and more or less anonymous audience, such as radio, television, films, newspapers, posters and books.

Medical approach to health education: Health education based on medical practice, that is, prescriptive and unidirectional, based on the conceptualisation of health as the absence of disease.

Meta-analysis: A set of (statistical) procedures designed to accumulate results across independent studies that address a related set of research questions.

Modelling: Learning from observing the actions of others and the consequences of their actions. See *Vicarious learning*.

Monitoring: Continuous evaluation to examine the ways in which programmes are implemented, including the processes of participation and collaboration, programme coverage, short-term impact of (parts of) the programme, problems, and possible solutions, to keep it on track and/or to improve the programme

Motivation: Internal state of desire which stimulates a person to a certain course of action or behaviour.

Motivation to comply: The individual inclination to live up to perceived expectations of others.

Multiple research methods: The use of more than one research method to obtain and compare results.

Multi-media approach: Communication approach making use of a combination of media in an intervention programme.

Multiple investigators: More than one investigator in one (research) programme. They bring their own specific domain of knowledge, information, as well as their own vision and standards, to programme development.

Multiple sources: Using different sources for collecting information (data) about one issue.

Network, electronic: A set of computers linked by cables, telephone line or via satellite connections that enables the exchange of information (data) between machines.

Network, personal: A set of direct and indirect social relations instrumental to the achievement of the goals of persons in the network.

Non-Governmental Organisation (NGO): An organisation which plays an intermediary role between the people and the government and/or tries to promote the welfare of a certain group of people. An NGO can be formed by members to improve their own situation, but also by outsiders who are trying to serve people's interests.

Norms: A set of values that define the range of acceptable and unacceptable attitudes and behaviours for members of a social unit. Norms specify certain rules or ways in which group members should behave. A norm can apply to a society (general norms), to certain groups or to a small group (such as a family, or school). In the second case it is called a group norm.

Normative beliefs: The individual's belief that each of a number of significant others expect him or her to act in a certain way.

Normative standards: Standards used in the formulation of objectives for health promotion programmes, where expectations are based on the level of performance achieved by other workers in programmes of a similar nature and designed for similar target groups.

Observability: The degree to which the results of an innovation are visible to others.

Opinion leader: A person who has a relatively large influence on the opinions of others in the group to which he or she belongs. Opinion leaders are seen as important contributors to the formation of public opinion about new ideas, situations, etc.

Organisation: Used here as a formal organisation: a formal group with explicit goals, a set of rules and procedures, and a clear division of tasks with set rights and duties. Every organisation also has an informal structure: the network of personal relations that arises spontaneously if individuals interact in a formal organisation.

Organisation structure: The network of interactions and relations between members of an organisation. The division of labour and power is regulated via the organisation structure.

Outcome expectancy: A person's estimate that a given behaviour will lead to certain outcomes.

Participation model of dialogue: Dialogue situations in which both the expert and the client play an active role in diagnosis of problems, in the analysis of possible causes, and in problem solving.

Participatory action research: Action research in which the researcher collaborates with all the others involved in a programme, including members of the target population See: *Action research*.

Participatory approach to health education: Health education is considered as a horizontal process of information exchange and interaction. The focus is on helping people to identify their own concerns and to gain the skills and confidence to act upon those concerns.

Perceived behavioural control: An individual's perception of how easy or difficult it is to perform a specific behaviour. See *Self-efficacy*.

Perception: The process by which individuals receive information or stimuli from their environment and transform it into psychological awareness.

Persuasive approach to health education: Individuals are encouraged to change their behaviour in a certain direction seen as conducive to health in the eyes of the expert.

Persuasive communication: A professional communication intervention to induce change in a voluntary behaviour, where such change is presumed to be of individual, public or collective benefit.

Policy: The set of objectives and rules guiding the activities of an organisation or an administration.

Post-test: The same instrument (usually a questionnaire) as used in the pre-test is administered to the same sample of the target population after interventions, in order to draw conclusions about the effectiveness of the interventions. See *Pre-test (2nd description)* and *Experimental research.*

Precontemplation stage: The stage at which individuals have no intention to change behaviour in the foreseeable future (Transtheoretical model of behaviour change).

Predisposing factors: Psychological or cognitive factors that influence the motivation of an individual or group to act.

Preliminary research: Research that focuses on diagnosis of the existing situation, the environmental and behavioural causes of health problems, and the determinants of these causes.

Preparation stage: Stage in which individuals have formed the intention to change behaviour (take action) in the immediate future, usually measured as the next month (Transtheoretical model of behaviour change).

Pre-test (1): Trial before introduction, as with health education publications and aids. Some people from the target group are shown the drafts. Their reactions are noted, and decisions are made as to whether the publications and aids are readable, entertaining and/or easily and correctly understood.

Pre-test (2): Instrument (usually a questionnaire) administered to a sample of the target population to provide baseline information for comparison with results on the post-test to enable conclusions to be drawn about the effectiveness of an intervention. See *Post-test* and *Experimental research.*

Prevention policy: Policy concerned with measures and activities aiming to prevent health problems.

Primary prevention: Aims to prevent health problems, diseases and accidents before they occur.

Professional coalitions: Coalitions which are formed by professional organisations, either in times of crisis or as a long-term approach to increasing their power and influence.

Programme development research: Research in relation to the development of health communication campaigns and action plans.

Programme objectives: Describe the specific activities that will be conducted in a programme in order to achieve the intervention objectives.

Propaganda: A conscious, systematic and organised effort to manipulate the decisions, actions and ideas of a large number of people, or to influence them with regard to a controversial subject, in a direction which is desirable from the point of view of the insights or interests of the propagandist.

Public relations: A communication function of the management of an organisation through which it tries to adapt, to alter, or to maintain the organisational environment for the purpose of achieving organisational goals.

Qualitative research: Research that collects and analyses data that can less easily or not at all be expressed in meaningful numbers, e.g. protocols of unstructured interviews, notes from observations, or minutes of meetings. Qualitative research focuses on processes and meanings.

Quantitative research: Research that collects and analyses data that can be expressed in numerical representations (quantity, amount, intensity, frequency) and that lend themselves to tests of statistical significance. Quantitative research focuses on the measurement and analysis of causal relations between variables.

Random sample: A sample from a population of which each person had an equal chance of being selected.

Rapid Participatory Appraisal: A research method to obtain information and understanding of characteristics of a social system (e.g. about the structure of a community), as well as to identify stakeholders. See *Stakeholders*.

Reinforcing factors: Positive or negative incentives that strengthen or inhibit behaviour (change).

Relative advantage of an innovation: The degree to which an innovation is perceived as better than the idea it supersedes.

Response costs: Costs involved in behaviour change (e.g. the loss of enjoyment associated with a risk behaviour). If the costs of the adaptive behaviour are perceived to be high, this will limit protection motivation.

Secondary prevention: Aims to limit the course of a disease or to reduce the risk of recurrence.

Selective acceptance: The tendency of people to accept messages more easily when the advocated position is in agreement with their own opinion.

Selective attention: The tendency of people to pay attention to information that is relevant to them, and to ignore information about subjects in which they are not interested.

Selective perception: The conscious or unconscious increase in attention to stimuli and information consistent with a person's attitudes or interests, or conscious or unconscious discounting of inconsistent stimuli.

Self-efficacy: An individual's perception of how easy or difficult it is to perform a specific behaviour. See *Perceived behavioural control*.

Self-help groups: Groups that are organised around a common problem of its participants, established to support each other in coping with, or solving, the problem. They are characterised by little or no involvement of professional helpers.

SMART criteria: Criteria for the design and specification of high quality objectives: Specific, Measurable, Agreed upon by all concerned, Realistic, Time bound.

Social norms: A set of values that define the range of acceptable and unacceptable attitudes and behaviours for members of a social unit. See *Norms*.

Stakeholders: People and organisations that have an interest or share in an issue. It includes both those who have an influence and those who are affected.

Subjective norm: The perception of an individual of the social pressures from important others to perform or not to perform a particular behaviour.

Survey research: Research aiming at a description of real life phenomena in terms of their content and extent, with the aid of a fixed schedule of questions. Data are often gathered from a representative sample of the whole population.

Synergy, principle of: The whole is more than the sum of its parts.

Synergy as a result of intersectoral collaboration: People, representing different institutions, with different backgrounds, different expertise and qualities, co-operate to achieve goals that they are unable to reach independently.

System of health care: Health services in relation to care, cure, and prevention.

Tailoring: Any combination of information or change strategies intended to reach one specific person (or a specific group), based on characteristics that are unique to that (those) person(s), relating to the outcome of interest, and derived from an individual assessment.

Target group; target population: A general indication of the group(s) at which interventions are aimed. It can refer to either (groups of) individuals or organisations.

Tertiary prevention: Aims to prevent existing health problems becoming worse, and to reduce disability due to health problems.

Theoretical standards: Standards used in the formulation of objectives for health promotion programmes, where expectations are derived from knowledge of relevant theory.

Threat appraisal: Assessment of a personal health threat, based on the perceived severity of, and the perceived vulnerability to, the threat.

Traditional research approach: Research based on the wish to discover, predict and control phenomena. It is typically related to experimental and survey research. Results from research are used 'to show', to find support for a hypothesis, or to show whether or not an intervention is effective. The researcher is an external observer. See *Biomedical research approach*.

Trialability: The extent to which an innovation may be tried out on a small scale.

Triangulation: Using more than one research approach to answer the same research question.

Validity evaluation: Assesses whether behavioural and environmental changes contribute to the achievement of the - higher level - health objective.

Vicarious learning: Learning from observing the actions of others and the consequences of those actions. See *Modelling*.

References

Aarts, M.N.C. (1998). *Een kwestie van natuur; een studie naar de aard en het verloop van communicatie over natuur en natuurbeleid.* Doctoral Dissertation. Wageningen: Wageningen Agricultural University.

Aas, H., Klepp, K.I., Laberg, J.C. & Aaro, L.E. (1995). Predicting adolescents' intentions to drink alcohol: Outcome expectancies and self-efficacy. *Journal of Studies on Alcohol, 56,* 293-299.

Agee, W.K., Ault, P.H. & Emery, E. (1988). Introduction to mass communications. New York: Harper Row. 9th edition.

Agudelo, C.A. (1983). Community participation in health activities: some concepts and appraisal criteria. In: Woelk, G.B. (1992). Cultural and structural influences in the creation of and participation in community health programmes. *Social Science and Medicine, 35(4),* 419-24.

Ajzen, I. (1985). From intentions to actions: a theory of planned behaviour. In: Kuhl, J., Beckmann, J. (Eds.). *Action control: From cognition to behavior.* Berlin: Springer Verlag.

Ajzen, I. (1988). *Attitudes, personality and behavior.* Milton Keynes: Open University Press.

Ajzen, I. (1991). The theory of planned behaviour. *Organizational Behavior and Human Decision Processes, 50,* 197-211.

Ajzen, I. & Fishbein, M. (1980). *Understanding attitudes and predicting social behaviour.* Englewood Cliffs, New York: Prentice Hall.

Ajzen, I. & Madden, T.J. (1986). Prediction of goal directed behaviour: attitudes, intentions and perceived behavioural control. *Journal of Experimental Social Psychology, 22,* 453-474.

Altman, D.G., Endres, J., Lorig, K., Howard-Pitney, B., & Rogers, T., (1991). Obstacles to and future goals of ten comprehensive community health promotion projects. *Journal of Community Health, 16,* 2999-314.

Amick, T.L. & Ockene, J.K. (1994). The role of social support in the modification of risk factors for cardiovascular disease. In: Shumaker, S.A. & Czajkowski, S.M. (Eds.). *Social support and cardiovascular disease.* New York: Plenum Press, 259-278.

Andersen, E.S., Grude, K.V. & Haug, T. (1995). *Goal directed project management: effective techniques and strategies.* London: Coopers & Lybrand.

Arnstein, S.R. (1971). Eight rungs on the ladder of citizen participation. In: Cahn, E.S., Passett, B.A. (Eds.). *Citizen participation: Effecting community change.* New York: Praeger Publishers, 69-91.

References

Ash, S.E. (1951). Effects of group pressure upon modification and distortion of judgements. In: Guetskow, H. (Ed.). *Groups, leadership and men.* Pittsburg PA: Carnegie Press.

Ash, S.E. (1956). Studies of independence and conformity: a minority of one against unanimous majority. *Psychological Monographs, 70, Whole No. 461.*

Ashton, J. (1988). Health promotion and the concept of community. In: Anderson, R., Davies, J.K., Kickbush, I. & Turner, J. (Eds.). *Health behaviour research and health promotion.* Oxford: Oxford Medical Publications.

Ashton, J. & Seymour, H. (1988). *The new public health.* Milton Keynes: Open University Press.

Ashworth, P. (1997). Breakthrough or bandwagon? Are interventions tailored to Stage of Change more effective than non-staged interventions? *Health Education Journal,* 56, 166-174.

Bandura, A. (1977). Self-efficacy: toward a unifying theory of behavior change. *Psychological Review,* 84, 191-215.

Bandura, A. (1982). Self-efficacy mechanism in human agency. *American Psychologist, 37,* 122-147.

Bandura, A. (1986). *Social foundations of thought and action; a social cognitive theory.* Englewood Cliffs, New York: Prentice Hall.

Bartholomew, L.K., Parcel, G.S., Kok, G. & Gottlieb, N. (2001) Intervention Mapping: Designing theory- and evidence based health promotion programs. New York: McGraw-Hill.

Batra, R. & Ray, M.L. (1983). Advertising situations: the implications of differential involvement and accompanying affect responses. In Harris, R.J. (Ed.). *Information processing research in advertising.* London: Lawrence Earlbaum Associates Publishers.

Beecher Stowe, H. (1852). *Uncle Tom's cabin.* Harvard Library Classics.

Behr, R. & Iyengar, S. (1985). Television news, real-world cues, and changes in the public agenda. *Public Opinion Quarterly, 49,* 38-57.

Berlo, D.K. (1960). *The process of communication.* New York: Holt, Rinehart and Winston.

Biddle, S.J. (1992). Exercise psychology. *Sport Science Review,* 1(2), 79-92.

Boonekamp, G.M.M., Vaandrager, H.W., Koelen, M.A. & Kennedy-Haynes, L. (1995). *Travelling through health promotion land. Guidelines for developing and sustaining health promotion programmes, derived form a European experience.* A publication from the SUPER-programme; IVESP-Valencia & Communication and Innovation Studies Wageningen Agricultural University.

Bouman, M. (1999). The Turtle and the Peacock: The entertainment education strategy on television. Doctoral Dissertation. Wageningen: Wageningen University.

Bracht, N. & Gleason, J. (1990). Strategies and structures for citizen partnerships. In: Bracht, N. (Ed.). *Health promotion at the community level*. London: Sage Publications.

Bracht, N., Kingsbury, L., & Rissel,. C. (1999). A five-stage community organization model for health promotion: empowerment and partnership strategies. In: Bracht, N. (Ed.). *Health promotion at the community level: New advances.* London: SAGE Publications. 2nd edition.

Bracht, N., & Tsouris, A. (1990). Principles and strategies of effective community participation. *Health Promotion International, 5,* 199-208.

Brewin, C.R. (1982). Adaptive aspects of self-blame in coping with accidental injury. In: Antaki, C. & Brewin, C.R. (Eds.). *Attributions and psychological change.* London: Academic Press.

Brewin, C.R. (1985). Depression and causal attributions: What is their relation? *Psychological Bulletin, 2,* 297-309.

Brug, J., Oenema, A. & Campbell, M. (2003). The past, the present and the future of computer tailored nutrition education. *The American Journal of Clinical Nutrition, 77,* 1028S-1034S.

Bruner, J.S. (1966). *Towards a theory of instruction.* Cambridge: Harvard University Press.

Butterfoss, F.D., Goodman, R.M. & Wandersman, A. (1993). Community coalitions for prevention and health promotion. *Health Education Research. Theory and Practice, 8,* 315 - 330.

Caburnay, C.A., Kreuter, M.W., Luke, D.A., Logan, R.A., Jacobsen, H.A., Reddy, V.C., Vempaty, A.R. & Zayed, H.R. (2003). The news on health behaviour: Coverage of diet, activity, and tobacco in local newspapers. *Health Education and Behaviour, 30,* 709-722.

Chaiken, S. (1987). The heuristic model of persuasion. In: Zanna, M.P., Olson, J.M., Herman, C.P. (Eds.). *Social influence: The Ontario symposium.* Vol 5,. Hillsdale, NJ: Erlbaum, 3-39

Chaiken, S. & Eagly, A.H. (1976). Communication modality as a determinant of message persuasiveness and message comprehensibility. *Journal of Personality and Social Psychology, 34,* 605-614.

Chavis, D. & Wandersman, A. (1990). Sense of community in the urban environment: A catalyst for participation and community development. *American Journal of Community Psychology, 18,* 55-77.

Children's Television Workshop (1998). Avaliable online at http://ctw.org. (retreived on January 15, 2001).

Clark, N.M., Baker, E.A., Chawla, A. & Maru, M. (1993). Sustaining collaborative problem solving: Strategies from a study in six Asian countries. *Health Education Research: Theory and Practice, 8,* 385-402.

References

CMPA Archive (1996). Assessing local news coverage of health issues. Center for Media and Public Affairs Archive. Available online at http://www.cmpa.com/archive/healthtv.htm (retreived on February 16, 2004).

Code of Ethics for the health education profession (2000). *Journal of Health Education, 31,* 216 - 218.

Contu, P. & Congiu, C. (1995). Health promotion through community participation: Project for Sardinia, Italy. In: Bruce, N., Springett, J., Hotchkiss, J., Scott-Samuel, J. (Eds.). *Research and change in urban community health.* Alderslot: Avebury Ashgate Publishing Limited, 359-368.

Cook, H.L., Goeppinger, J., Brunk, S.E. & Price, L.J. (1988). A reexamination of community participation in health: Lessons from three community health projects. *Family and Community Health, 11, (2),* 1-13.

Cook, T.D. & Campbell, D.T. (1979). *Quasi-experimentation: Design and analysis issues for field settings.* Chicago: Rand McNally College Publishing Company.

Cyber Atlas (2003). Active internet users by country. Available online at http://cyberatlas.internet.com/big_picture/geographics (retreived on February 13 2004).

De Haes, W.F.M., Voorham, A.J.J. & Mackenbach, J.P. (2002). Wijkgericht werken aan gezondheidsbevordering in vier achterstandswijken in Rotterdam. *TSG Tijdschrift voor Gezondheidswetenschappen, 80,* 425-430.

De Vries, H., Backbier, E., Kok, G., Dijkstra, M. (1995). The impact of social influence in the context of attitude, self-efficacy, intention, and previous behaviour as predictors of smoking onset. *Journal of Applied Social Psychology, 25,* 237-257.

DeVito, J.A. (1994). *Human communication: The basic course.* New York: Harper Collins College Publishers. 6th edition.

Dictionary of Marketing Terms (2004). Available online at http://www.marketingpower.com/live/mg-dictionary (retreived on January 6, 2004).

DiMatteo, M.R., DiNicola, D.D. (1982). *Achieving patient compliance. The psychology of the medical practitioner's role.* New York: Pergamon Press.

DiNicolla, D.D. & DiMatteo, R.M. (1984), Practitioners, patients, and compliance with medical regimes: A social psychological perspective. In: Baum, A., Tayler, S.E. & Singer, J.E. (Eds.). Handbook of psychology and health, Vol 4. 55-84. Hillsdale, NJ: Erlbaum.

Eagly, A.H.& Chaiken, S. (1993). *The psychology of attitudes.* Forth Worth, TX: Harcourt Brace Jovanovich.

Ecklund, L. (1999). *From citizen participation towards community empowerment.* Doctoral Dissertation. Tampere: School of Public health, University of Tampere.

Eiser, J.R. & Van Der Pligt, J. (1986). Smoking cessation and smokers' perceptions of their addiction. *Journal of Social and Clinical Psychology, 4,* 60-70.

Engel, J.F., Blackwell, R.D. & Miniard, P.W. (1986). *Consumer behaviour*. Chicago: The Dryden Press, 5th edition.

Feighery, E. & Rogers, T. (1989). *Building and maintaining effective coalitions.* Guide No. 12 in the series How-to Guides on Community Health Promotion. Palo Alto CA: Stanford Health Promotion Resource Center.

Festinger, L. (1957). *A theory of cognitive dissonance*. Stanford CA: Stanford University Press.

Finnegan, J.R. & Viswanath, K. (1999). Mass media and health promotion: Lessons learned with implications for public health campaigns. In: Bracht, N. (Ed.). *Health promotion at the community level.* London: SAGE Publications.

Finnegan, J.R., Viswanath, K., Kahn, K. & Hannan, P. (1993). Exposure to sources of heart disease prevention information: Community type and social group differences. *Journalism Quarterly, 70*, 560-584.

Fishbein, M. & Ajzen, I. (1975*). Belief, attitude, intention and behavior: An introduction to theory and research*. Reading MA: Addison-Wesley.

Fishbein, M. & Yzer, M.C. (2003). Using theory to design effective health behaviour interventions. *Communication Theory, 13*, 164-183.

Försterling, F. (1986). Attributional conceptions in clinical psychology. *American Psychologist, 41*, 275-285.

Försterling, F. (1988). *Attribution theory in clinical psychology*. New York: Wiley.

Frankish, C.J. & Green, L.W. (1994). Organisation and community change as the social scientific basis for disease prevention and health promotion policy. *Advances in Medical Sociology 4, 209-233.*

Frewer, L.J., Miles, S. & Marsh, E.R. (2002). The media and genetically modified foods: Evidence in support of social amplification of risk. *Risk Analysis, 22*, 701-711.

Gifford, S. (1996). Qualitative research: the soft option? *Health Promotion Journal of Australia*, 1996, 6, 58-61.

Godfrey, C. (2001). Economic evaluation of health promotion. In: Rootman, I., Goodstadt, M., Hyndman, B., McQueen, D.V., Potvin, L., Springett, J. & Ziglio, E. (Eds.). *Evaluation in health promotion: Principles and perspectives.* WHO Regional Publications, European Series, No. 92. Copenhagen: World Health Organisation.

Goodman, R.M., Wheeler, F.C. & Lee, P.R. (1995). Evaluation of the Heart to Heart project: Lessons from a community based chronic disease prevention project. *American Journal of Health Promotion*, 9, 443-455.

References

Goodstadt, M.S. Hyndman, B., McQueen, D.V., Potvin. L., Rootman, I. & Springett, J. Evaluation in health promotion: synthesis and recommendations. In: Rootman, I., Goodstadt, M., Hyndman, B., McQueen, D.V., Potvin, L., Springett, J. & Ziglio, E. (Eds.). *Evaluation in health promotion: Principles and perspectives.* WHO Regional Publications, European Series, No. 92. Copenhagen: World Health Organisation.

Goosen, S., Koelen, M., Langen, H., Berkouwer, L. & Van Schijndel. R. (2004). *Gezond AZC. Eindrapport van een pilot project gericht op gezondheidsbevordering in de centrale opvang van asielzoekers.* Utrecht: GGD Nederland, Landelijk Service Bureau MOA; Wageningen: Wageningen Universiteit, Leerstoelgroep Communicatie en Innovatie Studies.

Graham, K. & Bois, C. (1997). The complexity of roles in community action projects: The example of the evaluation of 'alternatives'. *Education and Programm Planning, 20,* 433-442.

Grandstaff, T.B. & Messerschmidt, D.A. (1995). *A manager's guide to the use of Rapid Rural Appraisal.* Bangkok, FAO/UNDP.

Green, L.W., Kreuter, M.W., Deeds, S.G. & Partridge, K.B. (1980). *Health education planning: A diagnostic approach.* Palo Alto: Mayfield Publishing Company.

Green, L.W., & Kreuter M.W., (1991). *Health promotion planning:An educational and environmental approach.* Palo Alto: Mayfield Publishing Company.

Green, L.W. & Lewis, F.M. (1986). *Measurement and evaluation in health education and health promotion.* Mayfield, Palo Alto, CA.

Green, L.W. & Reaburn, J.M. (1988). Health promotion: What is it? What will it become? *Health Promotion,* 3, 151-159.

Groot, A. (1999). *Stakeholder analysis tools.* International Course on Rural Extension. Wageningen: International Agricultural Centre Wageningen.

Haish, J., Ruch, G. & Haisch, I. (1985). Längerfristige Effecte attributionstherapeutiser Massnahmen bei Übergewichtigen: Auswirkungen eines Attributionestrainings auf Abnehmerfolg und Abbrecherquote bei einem 23 wöchigen Gewichtsreductions-Programm. *Psychotherapie und Medische Psychologie, 35,* 133-140.

Hanrahan, M. Prinsen, B. & de Graaf, Y. (1997). Mothers Inform Mothers: An innovative child care and development program in the Netherlands. In: Hanrahan, M. & Prinsen, B. (Eds.). *Community health, community care, community support.* Utrecht: Netherlands Institute of Care and Welfare (NIZW) Uitgeverij.

Harris, R.J. (1989). *A cognitive psychology of mass communication.* Hillsdale, NJ: Lawrence Erlbaum.

Hausenblas, H.A., Carron, A.V. & Mack, D.E. (1998). Application of the theories of reasoned action and planned behaviour to exercise behaviour: A meta-analysis. *Journal of Sport and Exercise Psychology, 19(1), 36-51.*

Hewstone, M. & Jaspers, J. (1983). A re-examination of the roles of consensus, consistency and distinctiveness: Kelley's cube revisited. *Britisch Journal of Social Psychology, 22,* 41-50.

Heymann, F. (1994). Educatieve voorlichting. In: Röling, N.G., Kuiper, D. & Janmaat, R. *Basisboek voorlichtingskunde.* Meppel: Boom.

Hilgard, E.R., Atkinson, R.C. & Atkinson, R.L. (1975). *Introduction to psychology.* New York: Harcourt Brace Jovanovich, Inc, 6th edition.

Horwath, C.C. (1999). Applying the transtheoretical model to eating behaviour change: Challenges and opportunities. *Nutrition Research Reviews, 12,* 281-317.

Hubey, J.H. (1985). Papers on community development (mimeo), Leeds Polytechnic. In: Tones, K., Tilford, S. (1994). *Health education: Effectiveness, efficiency and equity.* London: Chapman & Hall.

Janis, I.L. (1967). Effects of fear arrousal on attitude change: Recent developments in theory and experimental research. In: Berkowitz, L. (Ed.). *Advances in Experimental Social Psychology, 3.* New York: Academic Press.

Janz, N. & Becker, M.H. (1984). The health belief model: A decade later. *Health Education Quarterly, 11,* 1-47.

Judd, C.M., Smith, E.R., Kidder, L.H. (1991). *Research methods in social relations.* Forth Worth: Holt, Rhinehart and Winston.

Kasperson, R.E., Renn, O., Slovic, P., Brown, H.S., Emel, J., Goble, R., Kasperson, J.X. & Ratick, S. (1988). The social amplification of risk: A conceptual framework. *Risk Analysis, 8 (2),* 177-187.

Katz, D. & Kahn, R.L. (1978). *The social psychology of organizations,* New York: John Wiley & Sons. 2nd edition.

Kelly, H.H. (1967). Attribution theory in social psychology. In: Levine, D. (Ed.). *Nebraska Symposium on Motivation.* Lincoln: University of Nebraska Press.

Kelly, H.H. (1973). The process of causal attribution. *American Psychologist, 28,* 107-128.

Kelly, H.H. & Michela, J.L. (1980). Attribution theory and research. *Annual Review of Psychology, 31,* 457-501.

Kelly, J.A., St Lawrence, J.S., Diaz-Yolanda, E., Stevenson, L.Y., Hauth, A.C., Brasfield, T.L., Kalichman, S.C., Smith, J.E.& Andrew, M.E. (1991). HIV risk behaviour reduction following intervention with key opinion leaders of population: an experimental analysis. *American Journal of Public Health, 81,* 186-171.

Kessener, A.W. (1982). Gezondheidszorg, fictie of realiteit? *Medisch Contact, 37,* 335-338.

References

Kickbush, I. (1986). Health promotion: A global perspective. *Canadian Journal of Public Health, 77*, 321-326.

Klapper, J.T. (1960). *The effects of mass communication.* New York: Free Press.

Klepp, K.I., Halper, A. & Perry, C. (1986). The efficacy of peer leaders in drug abuse prevention. *Journal of School Health, 56*, 407-411.

Koelen, M.A. (1988). *Tales of logic: A self-presentational view on health related behaviour.* Doctoral Dissertation. Wageningen: Wageningen Agricultural University.

Koelen, M.A. (1992). Utilisation of knowledge in health promotion. In: Berlo, A. & Kiwitz-De Ruijter, Y. (Eds.). *Information in a healthy society; Health in the information society.* Knegsel: Akontes Publishing.

Koelen, M.A. (2000). *Evaluation of Super: The European food and shopping research.* Research report. Wageningen: Wageningen University.

Koelen, M.A. & Brouwers, T. (1990). Knowledge systems and public health. *Knowledge in Society: The International Journal of Knowledge Transfer, 3*, 50-57.

Koelen, M.A., Hielkema-de Meij, J.E. & Van der Sanden-Stoelinga, M.S.E. (2000). "Bottle it up - take a cup". The fight against nursing caries in the Netherlands: The campaign and its results. *International Journal of Health Promotion & Education, 38*, 47-53.

Koelen, M. & Martijn, C. (1994). Persuasieve voorlichting. In: Röling, N.G., Kuiper, D. & Janmaat, R. *Basisboek voorlichtingskunde.* Meppel: Boom.

Koelen, M.A. & Vaandrager, H.V. (1995). Health promotion requires innovative research techniques. In: Bruce, N., Springett, J., Hotchkiss, J. & Scott-Samuel, J. (Eds.). *Research and change in urban community health.* Alderslot: Avebury Ashgate Publishing Limited. p. 67-76.

Koelen, M.A. & Vaandrager, H.V. (1997). The Super-project: Five years of working according to the principles of health promotion. In: Bouman, L.I., Boonekamp, G.M.M. & Koelen, M.A. (Eds.) (1997). *Proceedings of the International Conference on Health Promotion and Nutrition,* organised by the European Super-project team in collaboration with the WHO Healthy Cities Project. Wageningen: Wageningen Agricultural University.

Koelen, M.A. & Vaandrager, H.V. (1999). Communicatieve veranderingsprocessen en onderzoek. In: Van Woerkum, C.M.J. & Van Meegeren, P. (1999). *Basisboek communicatie en verandering.* Amsterdam, Boom.

Koelen, M.A., Vaandrager, L., Colomer, C. (2001). Health promotion research: Dilemmas and challenges. *Journal of Epidemiology and Community Health, 55*, 257-262.

Koepsell, T.D., Diehr, P.H., Cheadle, A., Kristal, A. (1995). Invited Commentary: Symposium on Community Intervention Trials. *American Journal of Epidemiology 142 (6):* 594-599.

Krech, D., Crutchfield, R.S. & Ballachey, E.L. (1962). *Individual in society*. New York: McGraw-Hill.

Kreuter, M., Farrell, D., Olevitch, L. & Brennan, L. (2000). *Tailoring health messages: Customizing communication with computer technology*. Mahwah, NJ: Lawrence Erlbaum.

Kreuter, M.W. & Skinner, C.S. (2000). Tailoring: What's in a name. *Health Education Research, 15*, 1-4.

Kreuter, M.W., Lezin, N.A., Young, L.A. (2000). Evaluating community-based collaborative mechanisms: Implications for practitioners. *Health Promotion Practice, 1 (1)*, 49-63.

Krueger, R.A. (1991). *Focus groups: A practical guide for applied research*. London: Sage Publications.

Kumar, K. (Ed.) (1993). *Rapid Appraisal Methods*. Washington D.C.: World Bank.

Lamerichs, J. (2003). *Discourse of support: Exploring online discussions on depression*. PhD thesis. Wageningen: Wageningen University.

Landelijke Stichting Tegen Zinloos Geweld (2002). *Profielschets*. Available online at http://www.zinloosgeweld.nl (retreived on January 2, 2002).

LaPiere, R.T. (1934). Attitudes versus action. *Social Forces, 13*, 230-237.

Laverack, G. & Labonte, R. (2000). A planning framework for community empowerment goals within health promotion. *Health Policy and Planning, 15*, 255-262.

Leeuwis, C. & Van den Ban, A. (2004). *Communication for rural innovation:Rethinking agricultural extension*. Oxford: Blackwell Publishing.

Leippe, M.R. & Elkin, R.A. (1987). When motives clash: issue involvement and respons involvement as determinants of persuasion. *Journal of Personality and Social Psychology, 52*, 269-278.

Leventhal, H. & Cleary, P.D. (1980). The smoking problem: A review of research and theory in behavioural risk modification. *Psychological Bulletin, 88*, 370-405.

Lewin, K. (1953). Studies in group decision. In: Cartwright D, Zander A. (Eds.). *Group dynamics, research and theory*. Evanston: Row, Peterson Co.

Luepker, R.V., Murray, D.M., Jacobs, D.R. & Mittlemark, M.B. (1994). Community education for cardiovascular disease prevention: Risk factor changes in the Minnesota heart health program. *American Journal of Public Health, 84*, 1383-1393.

MacDonald, J.K. & Davies, G. (1998). Reflection and vision: Proving and improving the promotion of health. In: MacDonald, J.K. & Davies, G. *Quality, Evidence and effectiveness in health promotion*. London: Routledge.

Maslow, A.H. (1968). *Towards a psychology of being*. New York: Van Nostrand Reinhold.

References

McGuire, W.J. (1985). Attitudes and attitude change. In: Lindzey, G. & Aronson, E. (Eds.). *Handbook of social psychology*. New York: Random House, 233-246.

McMillan, D.W. & Chavis, D.M. (1986). Sense of community: a definition and theory. *Journal of Community Psychology, 14*, 6-23.

Mealand, J.G. & Haglund, B.J.A. (1999). Health promotion developments in the Nordic and related countries. In: Bracht, N. (Ed.). *Health promotion at the community level: New advances.* London: SAGE Publications.

Mechanic, D. (1999). Issues in promoting health. *Social Science & Medicine, 48*, 711-718.

Media Monitor (1997). 2000 Year in review: TV's leading news topics, reporters and political jokes. Volume XV, no 1. Available on http://www.cmpa.com/Mediamon/mm010201.htm (retreived on February 16, 2004)

Media Monitor (2001). Network news in the nineties: The top topics and trends of the decade, Volume XI, no 3. Available on http://www.cmpa.com/Mediamon/mm070897.htm (retreived on February 16, 2004)

Mendes, R. & Akerman, M. (2002). The challenge of project evaluation. In: Naerssen, T. Van & Barten, F. (Eds.). Healthy Cities in developing countries: Lessons to be learned. *Nijmegen Studies in Development and Cultural Change, 38.* Saarbrucken: Verlag für Entwicklungspolitik Saarbrucken GmbH.

Milio, N. (1997). Forging social responsibility in the world of the marketplace: moving governments to be modellers, market shapers and innovators. In: Bouman, L.I., Boonekamp, G.M.M. & Koelen, M.A. (Eds.) (1997). *Proceedings of the International Conference on Health Promotion and Nutrition,* organised by the European Super-project team in collaboration with the WHO Healthy Cities Project. Wageningen: Wageningen Agricultural University.

Millar, W.J. (1996). Reaching smokers with lower educational attainment. *Health Reports, 8*, 11-19.

Miller, W.L. & Crabtree, B.F. (1992). Primary care research: a multimethod typology and quality road map. In: Crabtree, B.F. & Miller, W.L. *Doing qualitative research.* Newbury Park: Sage Publications.

Mintzberg, H. (1983). *Power in and around organizations.* Prentice-Hall, Inc., Englewood Cliffs, N.J.

Molloy, B. (1997). The community mothers programme in Dublin. In: Hanrahan, M. & Prinsen, B. (Eds.). *Community health, community care, community support.* Utrecht: Netherlands Institute of Care and Welfare (NIZW) Uitgeverij.

Morgan, G. (1986). *Images of organization.* Beverly Hills: Sage Publications.

Narayan, D. (2002). *Empowerment and poverty reduction: A sourcebook.* Washington DC: The World Bank.

Northouse, P.G. & Northouse, L.L. (1992). *Health Communication: Strategies for Health Professionals*, Norwalk: Appleton and Lange, 2nd edition.

Nutbeam, D (1998a). *Health Promotion Glossary*. WHO/HPR/HEP/98.1. Geneva: World Health Organisation.

Nutbeam, D. (1998b). Evaluating health promotion-progress, problems and solutions. *Health Promotion International, 13(1), 27-44.*

Nutbeam, D. & Catfort, J. (1987). The Welsh heart programme: Progress, plans and possibilities. *Health Promotion International, 2,* 5-18.

Nutbeam, D. & Harris, E. (1998). *Theory in a nutshell. A practitioner's guide to commonly used theories and models in health promotion.* Sydney: University of Sydney, National Centre for Health Promotion, Department of Public health and Community Medicine.

Ockene, J., Ockene, I. & Kristellar, J. (1988). *The coronary artery smoking intervention study.* Worcester, MA: National Heart Lung Blood Institute.

Oei, T.P.S., Ferguson, S., Lee, N.K. (1998). The differential role of alcohol expectancies and drinking refusal self-efficacy in problem and non-problem drinkers. *Journal of Studies on Alcohol,* 59, 704-711.

Oenema, A., Brug, J. & Lechner, L. (2001). Web-based computer-tailored nutrition education: Results of a randomised controlled trial. *Health Education Research, 16,* 647-616.

Orvis, B.R., Cunningham, J.D. & Kelley, H.H. (1975). A closer examination of causal inference: The role of consensus, distinctiveness and consistency information. *Journal of Personality and Social Psychology, 32,* 605-616.

Pattison, S., Player, D. (1990). Health education: The political tensions. In: Doxiadis S. (Ed.). *Ethics in health education.* Chichester: John Wiley & Sons Ltd.

Petty, R.E. & Cacioppo, J.T. (1984). The effects of issue involvement on responses to argument quantity and quality: Central and peripheral routes to persuasion. *Journal of Personality and Social Psychology, 46,* 69-81.

Petty, R.E. & Cacioppo, J.T. (1986). The elaboration likelihood model of persuasion. In: Berkowitz, L. (Ed.). *Advances in experimental social psychology, 19.* New York: Academic Press, 123-205.

Pew Internet & American Life (2003). Internet health resources: Health searches and email have become more commonplace, but there is room for improvement in searches and overall internet access. Available online at http://www.pewinternet.org (retrieved on February 12, 2004).

Phelps, F.A., Mellandby, A.R., Crichton, N.J. & Tripp, J.H. (1994). Sex education: The effect of a peer programme on pupils (aged 13-14 years) and their peer leaders. *Health Education Journal,* 53, 127-139.

Pretty, J.N. (1995). *Regenerating agriculture:Policies and practice for sustainability and self-reliance.* London: Earthscan Publications Ltd.

Prochaska, J.O. & Velicer, W.F. (1997). The transtheoretical model of health behaviour change. *American Journal of Health Promotion, 12,* 38-48.

Prochaska, J.O., DiClemente, C.C. & Norcross, J.C. (1992). In search of how people change: Applications to addictive behaviour. *American Psychologist, 27,* 1102-1114.

Proost, M.D.C. (1993). De dagen van de landbouwvoorlichter zijn geteld: Over veranderingen in het beroep van de landbouwvoorlichter (The days of the agricultural extension agents have been counted: Changes in the extension profession). In: *Jaarboek Public Relations en Voorlichting.* The Hague: NGPR.

Puska, P., Nissinen, A. & Tuomilehto, J. (1985). The community-based strategy to prevent coronary heart disease: Conclusions from the ten years of the North Karelia project. *Annual Review of Public Health, 6,* 147-193.

Rakowski, W., Dube, C.E., Marcus, B.H., Prochaska, J.O., Velicer, W.F. & Abrams, D.B. (1992). Assessing elements of woman's decisions about mammography. *Health Psychology, 11,* 111-118.

Rappaport, J. (1985). The power of empowerment language. *Social Policy, 16,* 15-21.

Rappaport, J. (1987). Terms of empowerment; examplars of prevention: toward a theory for community psychology. *American Journal of Community Psychology, 15,* 121-148.

Reardon, K.K. (1991). *Persuasion in practice.* London: Sage Publications.

Rice, R.E. & Katz, J.E. (2001). *The internet and health communication. Experiences and expectations.* London: Sage.

Rifkin, S.B. (2000). Major issues arising from the literature review on participatory approaches to health improvement. In: Draper, A. & Hawdon, D. *Improving health through community participation: Concepts to commitment.* Proceedings of a Health Education Authority Workshop, 9-10 December, 1998, Leicester. London: Health Development Agency.

Rifkin, S.B., Lewando-Hundt, G. & Draper, A.K. (2000). *Participatory approaches in health promotion and health planning: A literature review.* London: Health Development Agency.

Rifkin, S.B., Muller, F. & Bichmann, W. (1988). Primary health care: On measuring participation. *Social Science Medicine, 26(9):* 931-40.

Rissel, C. (1994). Empowerment: The holy grail of health promotion? *Health Promotion International, 9,* 39-47.

Rogers, C.R. (1962). The interpersonal relationship: The core of guidance. *Harvard Educational Review, 32,* 416-529.

Rogers, E.M. (1983). *Diffusion of innovations.* New York: Free Press, 3rd edition.

Rogers, E.M. (1995). *Diffusion of innovations.* New York: Free Press, 4th edition.

Rogers, E.M. & Schoemaker, F.F. (1971). *Communication of innovations: A cross cultural approach.* New York: Free Press.

Rogers, R.W. (1975). A protection motivation theory of fear appeals and attitude change. *Journal of Psychology, 91*, 93-114.

Rogers, R.W. (1983). Cognitive and physiological processes in fear appeals and atitude change: A revised theory of protection motivation. In: Cacioppo, J.T. & Petty, R.E. (Eds.). *Social psychology: A source book*. New York: Guilford Press.

Rogner, O., Frey, D. & Haveman, D. (1985). *The relevance of cognitive factors on the recuperation process of accident patients*. Research report. Kiel: Department of Psychology, Christian Albrechts University.

Röling, N.G. (1988). *Extension science: Information systems in agricultural development*. Cambridge: Cambridge University Press.

Roncarati, D.D., Lefebvre, R.C. & Carleton, R.A. (1989). Voluntary involvement in community health promotion: The Pawtucket Heart Health Program. *Health Promotion, 4*, 11-18.

Rossi, P.H. & Freeman, H.E. (1993). *Evaluation, a systematic approach*. Newbury Park, California: Sage Publications, Inc. 5th edition.

Rossi, S.R., Rossi, J.S., Rossi-DelPrete, L.M., Prochaska, J.O., Banspach, S.W. & Carleton, R.A. (1994). A processes of change model for weight control for participants in community-based weight loss programs. *International Journal of the Addictions, 29*, 161-177.

Russel, M.A.H., Stapleton, J.A., Jackson, P.H., Hajek, P. & Belcher, M. (1987). District programme to reduce smoking: Effect of clinic supported brief intervention by general practitioners. *British Medical Journal, 295*, 1240-1244.

Ruwaard, D. Kramers, P.G.N., Van den Berg Jets, A. & Achterberg, P.W. (Eds.). (1994). *Public Health Status and Forecast: The health status of the Dutch population over the period 1950 - 2010*. RIVM. Den Haag: SDU-Uitgeverij.

Schaalma, H.P. (1995). *Planned development and evaluation of school-based AIDS/STD education*. Doctoral Dissertation. Maastricht: Maastricht University.

Schwarz, N. (1996). Survey research: Collecting data by asking questions. In: Semin, G.R. & Fiedler, K. (Eds.). *Applied social psychology*. Sage Publications, London.

Sears, D.O. & Freedman, J.L. (1971). Selective exposure to information: A critical review. In: Schramm, W. & Roberts, D.F. *The process and effects of mass communication*. Urbana: University of Illinois Press.

Seedhouse, D. (1992). *Ethics: The heart of health care*. Chichester: John Wiley and Sons Ltd.

Shapiro, C. & Varian, H.R. (1999). *Information rules. A strategic guide to the network economy*. Cambridge: Harvard Business School Press.

Sheeran, P. & Abraham, C. (1995). The health belief model. In: Conner, M. & Norman, P. (Eds.). *Predicting health behaviour*. Buckingham: Open University Press.

References

Sherif, C.W. (1980). Social values, attitudes, and involvement of the self. In: Page, M.M. (Ed.). *Nebraska Symposium on Motivation 1979: Beliefs, attitudes and values.* Lincoln: University of Nebraska Press, 1-64.

Sherif, C.W., Sherif, M. & Nebergall, R.E. (1965). *Attitude and attitude change: The social judgement-involvement approach.* Philadelphia: W.B. Saunders.

Sherif, M. & Hovland, C.I. (1961). *Social judgement: Assimilation and contrast effects in communication and attitude change.* New Haven, CT: Yale University Press.

Sherif, M. (1935). *The psychology of social norms.* New York: Harper & Row.

Siero, F.W. (1987). *Feedback en motivatie in de klas.* Doctoral Dissertation. Groningen: State University Groningen.

Simnett, I. (1995). *Managing health promotion: Developing healthy organizations and communities.* Chichester: John Wiley & Sons.

Singhal, A. & Rogers, E.M. (1999). *Entertainment education. A communication strategy for social change.* Mahwah, New Jersey: Lawrence Erlbaum Associates, Publishers.

Singhal, A. & Rogers, E.M. (2003). *Combating AIDS. Communication strategies in action.* London: Sage Publications.

Steptoe, A., Kerry, S., Rink, E. & Hilton, S. (2001). The impact of behavioral counseling on stage of change in fat intake, physical activity, and cigarette smoking in adults at increased risk of coronary heart disease. *American Journal of Public Health , 91 (2),* 265-269.

Steuart, G.W. (1965). Health behaviour and planned change: An approach to the professional preparation of the health education specialist. *Health Education Monographs, 20,* 3-26.

Stroebe, W. & De Wit, J. (1996). Health impairing behaviours. In: Semin, G.R. & Fiedler, K. *Applied Social Psychology.* London: Sage Publications.

Stroebe, W. (2000). *Social psychology and health.* Buckingham: Open University Press, 2nd edition.

Sullivan, M., Kone, A., Senturia, K.D., Chrisman, N.J., Ciske, S.J. & Krieger, J.W. (2001). Researcher and researched community perspectives: Towards bridging the gap. *Health Education and Behaviour, 28,* 130-149.

Sutton, S.R. (1982). Fear-arrousing communications: A critical examination of theory and research. In: Eiser, J.R. (Ed.). *Social psychology and behavioral medicine.* Chichester: John Wiley & Sons.

Tashakkori. A. & Teddlie C. (1998). Mixed methodology: Combining qualitative and quantitative approaches. *Applied Social Research Methods Series, 46.* London: Sage Publications.

Telch, M.J., Miller, L.M., Killen, J.D., Cooke, S. & Maccoby, N. (1990). Social influences approach to smoking prevention: The effects of a video tape delivery with and without same age peer leader participation. *Addictive Behaviours, 15,* 21-28.

Thompson, B. & Kinne, S. (1999). Social Change Theory: Applications to community health. In: Bracht, N. (Ed.). *Health promotion at the community level.* Newbury Park: Sage Publications.

Thompson, B. & Winner, C. (1999). Durability of community intervention programmes: Definitions, empirical studies, and strategic planning. In: Bracht, N. (Ed). *Health promotion at the community level.* Newbury Park: Sage Publications.

Tichenor, P.J., Donohue, G.A. & Olien, C.N. (1970). Mass media flow and differential growth in knowledge. *Public Opinion Quarterly, 34,* 159-170.

Tones, K. & Tilford, S. (1994). *Health education: Effectiveness, efficiency and equity.* London: Chapman & Hall.

Trauth, J.M., Ling, B.S., Weissfeld, J.L., Schoen, R.E. & Hayran, M. (2003). Using the transtheoretical models to stage screening behaviour for colorectal cancer. *Health Education and Behaviour, 30,* 322-336.

Trojan, A. (1989). Benefits of self-help groups: A survey of 232 members from 65 disease-related groups. *Social Science Medicine , 29,* 225-239.

Tschajanow, A. (1924). Die Sozialagronomie, Ihre Grundgedanken und Arbeitsmethoden. Berlin: Paul Parey (Original Moscow, 1917).

Turner, G. & Shepherd, J. (1999). A method in search of a theory: Peer education and health promotion. *Health Education Research, 14,* 235-247.

Tuveri, R. & Koelen, M. (1998). *Intersectoral collaboration in Eindhoven: From theory to practice.* Research Report. Wageningen: Wageningen Agricultural University.

Vaandrager, H.W. (1995). *Constructing a healthy balance: Action and research ingredients to facilitate the process of health promotion.* Doctoral Dissertation. Wageningen: Agricultural University, Communication and Innovation Studies.

Vaandrager, L. & Koelen, M.A. (1997). Consumer involvement in nutritional issues: The role of information. *The American Journal of Clinical Nutrition. 65, 6(S).*

Vaandrager, H.W., Koelen, M.A., Ashton. J.R. & Colomer Revuelta, C. (1994). A four-step health promotion approach for changing dietary patterns in Europe. *European Journal of Public Health,* 3,193-198.

Van de Velde, F.W., Van der Pligt, J. & Hooykaas, C. (1994). Perceiving AIDS-related risks: Accuracy as a function of differences in actual risk. *Health Psychology, 23,* 25-33.

Van den Ban, A.W. & Hawkins H.S. (1996). Agricultural extension. Oxford: Blackwell Science. 2nd edition.

References

Van Ginneken, J. (1996). *Brein-bevingen. Snelle omslagen in opinie en communicatie.* Amsterdam: Boom.

Van Knippenberg, A. & Koelen, M.A. (1985). Attributional self-presentation and information available to the audience. *European Journal of Social Psychology, 15,* 249-261.

Van Woerkum, C.M.J. (1999). Massamediale communicatie. In: Van Woerkum, C.M.J. & Van Meegeren, P. (1999). *Basisboek communicatie en verandering.* Amsterdam, Boom.

Van Woerkum, C., Kuiper, D. & Bos, E. (1999). *Communicatie en innovatie: Een inleiding.* Alphen aan den Rijn: Samsom.

Verderber, R.F. (1996). *Communicate!* Belmont: Wadsworth Publishing Company.

Verheijden, M.W., Van der Veen, J.E., Van Zadelhoff, W.M., Bakx, J.C., Koelen, M.A., Van den Hoogen, H.J.M., Van Weel, C. & Van Staveren, W.A. (2003). Nutrition guidance in Dutch family practice: Behavioral determinants of reduction of fat consumption. *American Journal of Clinical Nutrition 77,* 1058S-1064S.

Von Bertalanffy, L. (1968). *General systems theory: Foundations, development, applications.* New York: Braziller.

Voorham, A.J.J. (2003). *Gezondheidsbevordering voor-en-door de doelgroep. Theoretische onderbouwing en evaluatie bij migranten en ouderen.* PhD thesis. Rotterdam: GGD Rotterdam e.o.

Voorham, A.J.J., De Haes, W.F.M., & Mackenbach, J.P. (2002). Wijkgericht werken aan gezondheidsbevordering in vier achterstandswijken in Rotterdam: Leerpunten uit de praktijk. *TSG Tijdschrift voor Gezondheidswetenschappen, 80,* 431-435.

Wagemakers, A. & Koelen, M. (2001). *Samenwerken aan gezondheid in de buurt: Een jaar verder. Actiebegeleidend onderzoek in Eindhoven.* Verslag van de tweede evaluatieronde. Wageningen: Wageningen Universiteit, Communicatie en Innovatie Studies.

Wagemakers, A. (2000). *Samenwerken aan gezondheid in de buurt. Actiebegeleidend onderzoek in Eindhoven.* Verslag van de eerste evaluatieronde. Wageningen: Wageningen Universiteit, Communicatie en Innovatie Studies.

Wallbott, H.G. (1996). Social psychology and the media. In: Semin, G.R & Fiedler, K. (Eds.). *Applied social psychology.* London: Sage Publications.

Wallerstein N (1992). Powerlessness, empowerment, and health: implications for health promotion programs. *American Journal of Health Promotion, 6,* 197-205.

Wallerstein, N. (2000). A participatory evaluation model for healthier communities: Developing indicators for New Mexico. *Public Health Reports,* 115, 199-204

Wallerstein, N. (1999). Power between evaluator and community: Research relationships within New Mexico's healthier communities. *Social Science & Medicine,* 49, 39-53.

Wandersman, A. & Giamartino, G. (1980). Community and individual difference characteristics as influences on initial participation. *American Journal of Community Psychology, 2,* 217-229.

Watzlawick, P., Beavin, J.H. & Jackson, D.D. (1967). *Pragmatics of human communication: A study of interactional patterns, pathologies, and paradoxes.* New York: Norton.

Weick, K.E. (1979). *The social psychology of organizing.* Addison-Wesley Publishing Company, London.

Weijters, J. & Koelen, M. (2002). *Samenwerken aan gezondheid in de buurt. Actiebegeleidend onderzoek in Eindhoven.* Verslag van de vierde evaluatieronde. Wageningen: Wageningen Universiteit, Communicatie en Innovatie Studies.

Weiner, B. (1986). *An attributional theory of motivation and emotion.* New York: Springer Verlag.

Weiner, B., Frieze, I., Kukla, A., Reed, L., Rest, S. & Rosenbaum, R.M. (1971). Perceiving the causes of success and failure. In: Jones, E.E., Kanouse, D.E., Kelley, H.H., Nisbett, R.E., Valins, S. & Weiner, B. (Eds.). *Attribution: Perceiving cause of behaviour.* Morristown, NJ: General Learning Press.

Weinstein, N.D. (1987). Unrealistic optimism about susceptibility to health problems: Conclusions from a community-wide sample. *Journal of Behavioural Medicine, 10,* 481-500.

Weinstein, N.D. (1988). The precaution adoption process. *Health Psychology, 7,* 355-386.

Weinstein, N.D. (1989). Optimistic biases about personel risks. *Science, 246,* 1232-1233.

Welch-Cline, R. (1999). Communication in social support groups. In: Frey, L., Gouran, D. & Poole, S. (Eds.). *Handbook of small group communication.* Newbury Park: Sage.

Whyte, F.W., Greenwood, D.J., Lazes, P. (1991). Participatory action research: Through practice to science in social research. In: Whyte W. (Ed.). *Participatory action research.* Newbury Park: SAGE Publications Inc.

Wilmot, W.W. (1987). *Dyadic communication.* New York: Random House. 3rd edition.

Windahl, S., Signitzer, B. & Olson, J.T. (1991). *Using communication theory: An introduction to planned change.* London: Sage.

Withag, J.G. (1990). Winst en wetenschap: Communicatie en overleg in een machinebureaucratie. Doctoral Thesis. Wageningen: Wageningen Agricultural University.

World Bank (1998). *World development report 1998/1999. Knowledge for development.* New York: Oxford University Press.

World Health Organisation (1978). *Alma Ata 1977. Primary Health Care.* Geneva: WHO, UNICEF.

References

World Health Organisation (1981). *Global Strategy for Health For All by the Year 2000*. Geneva: WHO.

World Health Organisation Europe (1981). *Regional Strategy for Attaining Health for All by the year 2000*. EUR/RC 3018. Rev. 1. Copenhagen: WHO.

World Health Organisation (1986). *Ottawa Charter of health promotion*. Copenhagen: WHO.

World Health Organization (1991). *Improving urban health. Guidelines for rapid appraisal to assess community health needs. A focus on health improvements for low income urban areas*. WHO, Geneva.

World Health Organisation (1998). *Resolution of the World Health Assembly on Health promotion*. World Health Assembly. *Document A51/5*: Health for All policy for the twenty-first century. Geneva: WHO.

World Health Organisation Europe (1998). *Health 21. An introduction to the health for all policy framework for the WHO European Region*. European Health for All Series No. 5. Copenhagen: WHO.

World Health Organisation (2002). *The World Health Report 2002: Reducing risks, promoting healthy life*. Geneva: World Health Organisation.

Yeo, M. (1993). Toward an ethic of empowerment for health promotion. *Health promotion International, 8*, 225 - 235.

Zakus, J.D.L. & Lysack, C.L. (1998). Revisiting community participation. *Health Policy and Planning, 13 (1)*, 1-12.

Zimbardo, P.G. & Leippe, M.R. (1991). *The psychology of attitude change and social influence*. Boston: McGraw-Hill.

Guide for further reading

Chapter 2

Nutbeam, D. (1998). *Health Promotion Glossary*. WHO/HPR/HEP/98.1. Geneva: World Health Organisation.

World Health Organisation (1986). *Ottawa Charter of Health Promotion*. Copenhagen: World Health Organisation.

World Health Organisation Europe (1998). *Health 21. An introduction to the health for all policy framework for the WHO European Region*. European Health for All Series No. 5. Copenhagen: WHO.

Chapter 3

Marks, D.F., Murray, M., Evans, B. & Willig, C. (2000). *Health psychology: Theory, research and practice*. London: Sage Publications.

Smith, E.R. & Mackie, D.M. (2000). *Social psychology*. Philadelphia: Psychology Press, 2nd edition.

Stroebe, W. (2000). *Social psychology and health*. Buckingham: Open University Press, 2nd edition.

Chapter 4

Rogers, E.M.. (2003). *Diffusion of innovations*. New York: Free Press, 5th edition.

Chapter 5

DeVito, J.A. (1994). *Human communication: The basic course*. New York: Harper Collins College Publishers. 6th edition.

Verderber, R.F. (1996). *Communicate!* Belmont: Wadsworth Publishing Company.

Zimbardo, P.G. & Leippe, M.R. (1991). *The psychology of attitude change and social influence*. Boston: McGraw-Hill.

Chapter 6

Maibach, E. & Parrott, R.I. (1995). *Designing health messages: Approaches from communication theory and public health practice*. Thousand Oaks: Sage Publications.

Singhal, A. & Rogers, E.M. (1999). *Entertainment education. A communication strategy for social change*. Mahwah, New Jersey: Lawrence Erlbaum Associates, Publishers.

Singhal, A. & Rogers, E.M. (2003). *Combating AIDS. Communication strategies in action*. London: Sage Publications.

Windahl, S., Signitzer, B. & Olson, J.T. (1991). *Using communication theory: An introduction to planned change*. London: Sage.

Chapter 7

Bracht, N. (Ed) (1999) *Health promotion at the community level. New advances.* London: Sage Publications, 2nd edition.

Leeuwis, C. With contributions of Van den Ban, A. (2004). *Communication for rural innovation: Rethinking agricultural extension*. Oxford: Blackwell Publishing.

Narayan, D. (2002). *Empowerment and poverty reduction: A sourcebook*. Washington DC: The World Bank.

Rifkin, S.B., Lewando-Hundt, G. & Draper, A.K. (2000). *Participatory approaches in health promotion and health planning: A literature review*. London: Health Development Agency.

Chapter 8

Bartholomew, L.K., Parcel, G.S., Kok, G. & Gottlieb, N. (2001). *Intervention Mapping: Designing theory- and evidence based health promotion programs*. New York: McGraw-Hill.

Bracht, N (Ed) (1999) *Health promotion at the community level*. New advances. 2nd edition, London: Sage Publications.

Green L.W., & Kreuter M.W., (1999). *Health promotion planning: an educational and ecological approach*. Mountain View, CA: Mayfield Publishing, 3rd edition.

Tones, K. & Tilford, S. (2001). *Health promotion: effectiveness, efficiency and equity*. London: Nelson Thornes, 3rd edition.

Chapter 9:

Judd, C.M., Smith, E.R., Kidder, L.H. (1991). *Research methods in social relations.* Forth Worth: Holt, Rhinehart and Winston.

Rootman, I., Goodstadt, M. Hyndman, B., McQueen, D.V. Potvin, L., Springett, J. & Ziglio (2001). *Evaluation in health promotion: Principles and perspectives.* WHO Regional Publications, European Series, No. 92. Copenhagen: World Health Organisation.

Rossi, P.H. & Freeman, H.E. (1993). *Evaluation, a systematic approach*. Newbury Park, California: Sage Publications, Inc., 5th edition.

Chapter 10

Andersen, E.S., Grude, K.V. & Haug, T. (1995). *Goal directed project management: effective techniques and strategies*. London: Coopers & Lybrand.

Davies, A. (1997). *Managing for change: How to run community development projects*. London: Intermediate Technology Publications.

Simnett, I. (1995). *Managing health promotion: Developing healthy organizations and communities.* Chichester: John Wiley & Sons.

Index

G

goal directed project management – 215
group discussions – 100
group method – 120
    -advantages – 125
    -disadvantages – 125
    -effects of – 122

H

health – 26
    -care policy – 39
    -education – 30
    -education, definition – 32
    -literacy – 32
    -policies – 37
    -promotion – 33, 38
    -promotion ethics – 225
    -protection – 38
    -the role of professionals – 36
health belief model – 60
Health for All by the Year 2000 – 39
Health for All in the 21st century – 40
healthy public policies – 37
hierarchy of needs – 26, 150
horizontal communication flow – 212
hybrid media – 100, 126
    -potential qualities – 129
hypes – 113

I

ICT – 126
identification of resources – 172
immanent change – 143
implementation – 157, 177
importance of a behaviour – 163
individual change – 71
induced immanent change – 144
informational communication – 95
informational social influence – 67
innovation – 71

    -adoption of – 71
    -characteristics – 84
innovators – 80
intention to perform behaviour – 55
intermediate indicators – 195
internal attribution – 50
internal communication – 211
internal validity – 195
    -diffusion of treatments – 197
    -history – 196
    -instrumentation – 197
    -maturation – 196
    -mortality – 197
    -selection – 197
    -testing – 197
    -threats to – 196
interpersonal communication – 100, 130
intersectoral
    -action – 139
    -collaboration – 135, 138
    -collaboration, barriers to – 151
    -policy – 39
intervention mix – 170
intervention objectives – 167
involvement – 105, 145
involving population – 34, 64

L

laggards – 81
language – 99
late majority – 80
latitude of acceptance – 104
latitude of non-commitment – 105
latitude of rejection – 104
Law of Effect – 46
leadership – 214
leadership structure of an
    organisation – 214
leaflets – 111
learning – 45